Use of Biologics for Foot and Ankle Surgery

Editor

ADAM S. LANDSMAN

CLINICS IN PODIATRIC MEDICINE AND SURGERY

www.podiatric.theclinics.com

Consulting Editor

THOMAS J. CHANG

July 2018 • Volume 35 • Number 3

ELSEVIER

1600 John F. Kennedy Boulevard • Suite 1800 • Philadelphia, Pennsylvania, 19103-2899

http://www.theclinics.com

CLINICS IN PODIATRIC MEDICINE AND SURGERY Volume 35, Number 3
July 2018 ISSN 0891-8422, ISBN-13: 978-0-323-61289-0

Editor: Lauren Boyle
Developmental Editor: Sara Watkins

Clinics in Podiatric Medicine and Surgery (ISSN 0891-8422) is published quarterly by Elsevier Inc., 360 Park Avenue South, New York, NY 10010-1710. Months of issue are January, April, July, and October. Business and Editorial Offices: 1600 John F. Kennedy Blvd., Ste. 1800, Philadelphia, PA 19103-2899. Customer Service Office: 3251 Riverport Lane, Maryland Heights, MO 63043. Periodicals postage paid at New York, NY and additional mailing offices. Subscription prices are $294.00 per year for US individuals, $544.00 per year for US institutions, $100.00 per year for US students and residents, $382.00 per year for Canadian individuals, $657.00 for Canadian institutions, $439.00 for international individuals, $657.00 per year for international institutions and $220.00 per year for Canadian and foreign students/residents. To receive student/resident rate, orders must be accompanied by name of affiliated institution, date of term, and the *signature* of program/residency coordinator on institution letterhead. Orders will be billed at individual rate until proof of status is received. Foreign air speed delivery is included in all *Clinics* subscription prices. All prices are subject to change without notice. POSTMASTER: Send address changes to *Clinics in Podiatric Medicine and Surgery*, Elsevier Health Sciences Division, Subscription Customer Service, 3251 Riverport Lane, Maryland Heights, MO 63043. **Customer Service: 1-800-654-2452 (US). From outside of the US, call 314-447-8871. Fax: 314-447-8029. E-mail: JournalsCustomerService-usa@elsevier.com (for print support); JournalsOnlineSupport-usa@elsevier.com (for online support).**

Reprints. For copies of 100 or more of articles in this publication, please contact the Commercial Reprints Department, Elsevier Inc., 360 Park Avenue South, New York, NY 10010-1710. Tel.: 212-633-3874; Fax: 212-633-3820; E-mail: reprints@elsevier.com.

Clinics in Podiatric Medicine and Surgery is covered in *MEDLINE/PubMed (Index Medicus) and EMBASE/Excerpta Medica.*

Contributors

CONSULTING EDITOR

THOMAS J. CHANG, DPM
Clinical Professor and Past Chairman, Department of Podiatric Surgery, California College of Podiatric Medicine, Faculty, The Podiatry Institute, Redwood Orthopedic Surgery Associates, Santa Rosa, California, USA

EDITOR

ADAM S. LANDSMAN, DPM, PhD, FACFAS
Chief, Division of Podiatric Surgery, Assistant Professor, Department of Surgery, Cambridge Health Alliance, Harvard Medical School, Cambridge, Massachusetts, USA

AUTHORS

HASEEB AHMAD, DPM
Residency Program, Veterans Administration Hospital, East Orange, New Jersey, USA

JOEL ANG, DPM, MS
2nd Year Resident, Podiatric Medicine and Surgery, Department of Surgery, Cambridge Health Alliance, Clinical Fellow in Surgery, Harvard Medical School, Cambridge, Massachusetts, USA

DARRELL BARNHART, BS
Vice President, Kent Imaging, Calgary, Canada

LAURA BOHMAN, DPM, AACFAS
Podiatric Surgeon, Podiatry Associates of Cincinnati, Cincinnati, Ohio, USA

JENNIFER BUCHANAN, DPM
Attending Physician, Division of Podiatric Surgery, Cambridge Health Alliance, Cambridge, Massachusetts, USA

SAMEEP CHANDRANI, DPM
Residency Program, Veterans Administration Hospital, East Orange, New Jersey, USA

AMANDA CROWELL, DPM
Ocean County Foot & Ankle Surgical Associates, P.C., Toms River, New Jersey, USA

ROBERT C. FLOROS, DPM, FACFAS
Ocean County Foot & Ankle Surgical Associates, P.C., Toms River, New Jersey, USA

NAJWAH HAYMAN, DPM
Cambridge Health Alliance, Cambridge, Massachusetts, USA

KELLI L. ICEMAN, DPM
PGY-3, Podiatric Medicine and Surgery Resident, Gundersen Medical Foundation, La Crosse, Wisconsin, USA

JASON A. KAYCE, DPM
Paradise Valley Foot and Ankle, Phoenix, Arizona, USA

ADAM S. LANDSMAN, DPM, PhD, FACFAS
Chief, Division of Podiatric Surgery, Assistant Professor, Department of Surgery, Cambridge Health Alliance, Harvard Medical School, Cambridge, Massachusetts, USA

ROBIN LENZ, DPM
Ocean County Foot & Ankle Surgical Associates, P.C., Toms River, New Jersey, USA

CHIH-KANG DAVID LIOU, DPM
2nd Year Resident, Podiatric Medicine and Surgery, Department of Surgery, Cambridge Health Alliance, Clinical Fellow in Surgery, Harvard Medical School, Cambridge, Massachusetts, USA

MEGAN LUBIN, DPM, MS, FACFAS
Ocean County Foot & Ankle Surgical Associates, P.C., Toms River, New Jersey, USA

MARK K. MAGNUS, DPM
PGY-3, Podiatric Medicine and Surgery Resident, Gundersen Medical Foundation, La Crosse, Wisconsin, USA

GARRETT MELICK, DPM
Cambridge Health Alliance, Cambridge, Massachusetts, USA

RUSSELL D. PETRANTO, DPM, FACFAS
Ocean County Foot & Ankle Surgical Associates, P.C., Toms River, New Jersey, USA

DARELLE A. PFEIFFER, DPM, FAPWCA, FACFAS
Ocean County Foot & Ankle Surgical Associates, P.C., Toms River, New Jersey, USA

MELISSA K. RICHARDSON, MD
Medical Director, Bon Secours St Francis Wound Healing Center, Greenville, South Carolina, USA

THOMAS S. ROUKIS, DPM, PhD, FACFAS
Attending Staff, Orthopaedic Center, Gundersen Healthcare System, La Crosse, Wisconsin, USA

ELAINE W. RUSH, RN, BS, CWOCN
Quality and Research Coordinator, Bon Secours St Francis Wound Healing Center, Greenville, South Carolina, USA

HARRY P. SCHNEIDER, DPM
Residency Director, Podiatric Medicine and Surgery, Department of Surgery, Cambridge Health Alliance, Assistant Professor of Surgery, Harvard Medical School, Cambridge, Massachusetts, USA

MICHAEL SOWA, PhD
Chief Science Officer, Kent Imaging, Calgary, Canada

KERIANNE SPIESS, DPM
Ocean County Foot & Ankle Surgical Associates, P.C., Toms River, New Jersey, USA

MICHAEL H. THEODOULOU, DPM, FACFAS
Podiatric Surgeon, Department of Surgery, Cambridge Health Alliance, Instructor of Surgery, Harvard Medical School, Cambridge, Massachusetts, USA

MICHAEL A. TOWLER, MD, FACS
Surgical Director, Bon Secours St Francis Wound Healing Center, Greenville, South Carolina, USA

CALVIN L. WILLIAMS, PhD
Professor, Department of Mathematical Sciences, Center for Excellence in Mathematics and Science Education, Clemson University, Clemson, South Carolina, USA

Contents

Foreword: Use of Biologics in Foot and Ankle Surgery xi

Thomas J. Chang

Preface: Use of Biologics for Foot and Ankle Surgery xiii

Adam S. Landsman

Complications Following Allograft and Xenograft Resurfacing of the First Metatarsal Head: A Case Series 271

Jason A. Kayce, Jennifer Buchanan, and Adam S. Landsman

Ten cases using decellularized allografts and xenografts for the purpose of resurfacing the first metatarsal head are reviewed in this article. Although most of the cases were performed without any post-operative complications, the focus of this series is on 2 of the 3 cases in which destruction of the first metatarsal head was observed postoperatively owing to a foreign body reaction and severe degeneration within the metatarsal head. A salvage procedure using a silicone total joint to replace the damaged surface is shown. Cystic changes present preoperatively, and their role in subsequent failure is examined.

Allograft Cartilage Replacements 281

Michael H. Theodoulou and Laura Bohman

The body's abillty to repair injured articular cartilage is poor because of the inherent physiology of cartilage. Joint arthritis, whether through injury or increasing age, is a prevalent condition. Treatment of an articular cartilage injury may include arthroplasty, fusion, or repair. A popular pathway of treatment in a salvageable joint is often to avoid donor site morbidity and place increased effort to reestablish native cartilage with the use of allografts. This article discusses current research on acellular and cellular allografts for articular cartilage restoration.

Living Cryopreserved Bone Allograft as an Adjunct for Hindfoot Arthrodesis 295

Mark K. Magnus, Kelli L. Iceman, and Thomas S. Roukis

Hindfoot arthrodesis is a frequently performed procedure by foot and ankle surgeons. The relatively high nonunion rate associated with these procedures has led surgeons to use adjunctive bone graft to help augment osseous union. Cellular bone allografts are a specific type of graft that incorporates osteoconductive, osteoinductive, and osteogenic properties while also eliminating the common disadvantages of autografts and traditional allografts. This article discusses the role of cellular bone allografts in hindfoot arthrodesis procedures, a review of the current literature, and a comparison of available products.

Special Article

Randomized, Prospective, Blinded-Enrollment, Head-To-Head Venous Leg Ulcer Healing Trial Comparing Living, Bioengineered Skin Graft Substitute (Apligraf) with Living, Cryopreserved, Human Skin Allograft (TheraSkin) **357**

Michael A. Towler, Elaine W. Rush, Melissa K. Richardson, and Calvin L. Williams

Chronic venous leg ulcers are responsible for significant morbidity and health care costs worldwide. This pilot study evaluated the effectiveness of 2 biologically active grafts, TheraSkin and Apligraf, in conjunction with compression therapy. The study, not industry sponsored, was designed and conducted as a prospective, head-to-head, single-site, randomized clinical trial to assess differences in healing rates, adverse outcomes, and treatment costs. The healing rates were different but not statistically significant, there were no adverse outcomes, and TheraSkin averaged $2495.33 and Apligraf averaged $4316.67 per subject. This suggests that TheraSkin may provide equivalent or superior outcomes to Apligraf while reducing costs.

CLINICS IN PODIATRIC MEDICINE AND SURGERY

FORTHCOMING ISSUES

October 2018
Innovations in Foot and Ankle Surgery
Guido A. LaPorta, *Editor*

January 2019
Perioperative Considerations in the Surgical Patient
Jeffrey Shook, *Editor*

April 2019
Current Perspectives on Management of Calcaneal Fractures
Thomas S. Roukis, *Editor*

RECENT ISSUES

April 2018
Advanced Techniques in the Management of Foot and Ankle Trauma
Justin J. Fleming, *Editor*

January 2018
New Technologies in Foot and Ankle Surgery
Stephen A. Brigido, *Editor*

October 2017
Surgical Advances in Ankle Arthritis
Alan Ng, *Editor*

RELATED INTEREST

Foot and Ankle Clinics, September 2017 (Vol. 22, No. 3)
The Flatfoot: Pearls and Pitfalls
Kent Ellington, *Editor*
Available at: http://www.foot.theclinics.com/

Foreword

Use of Biologics in Foot and Ankle Surgery

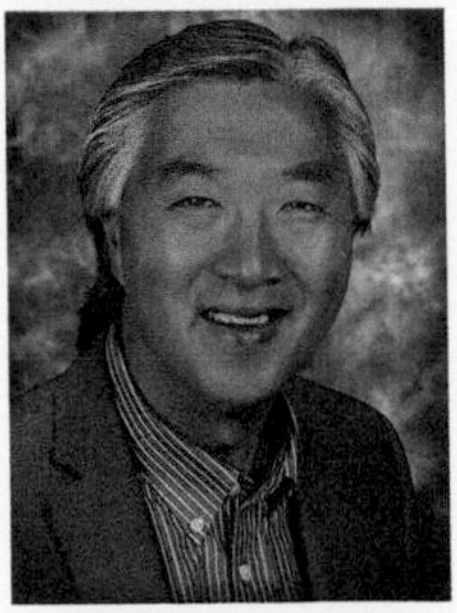

Thomas J. Chang, DPM
Consulting Editor

Time flies… here we are on the third issue of *Clinics in Podiatric Medicine and Surgery* in 2018. Biologics have been a special interest of mine for most of my career. This started with demineralized bone matrixes (DBMs) in the 1990s and then moved onto bone morphogenic proteins (BMPs) in the 2000s, and now we have mesenchymal stem cells (MSCs) and bone marrow aspirates (BMAs), which essentially convert bone allograft products into bone autograft equivalents. Each decade has provided tremendous advances on how to create a better environment in our difficult clinical scenarios. We are constantly looking for the Holy Grail to enhance our wound healing, soft tissue injuries, and bone procedures.

I am pleased Dr Landsman has taken on this issue. As a bioengineer and surgeon, he has tremendous insight into the problems we all face, and the cutting-edge research available to solve these problems. There are great articles in this issue that cover all the pertinent tissue types we deal with in the surgical realm. I thank him and the authors for the shared knowledge.

I hope you enjoy this timely topic of Biologics 2018.

Thomas J. Chang, DPM
Department of Podiatric Surgery
California College of Podiatric Medicine
The Podiatry Institute
Redwood Orthopedic Surgery Associates
208 Concourse Boulevard
Santa Rosa, CA 95403, USA

E-mail address:
thomaschang14@comcast.net

Clin Podiatr Med Surg 35 (2018) xi
https://doi.org/10.1016/j.cpm.2018.03.002
0891-8422/18/© 2018 Published by Elsevier Inc.
podiatric.theclinics.com

Preface
Use of Biologics for Foot and Ankle Surgery

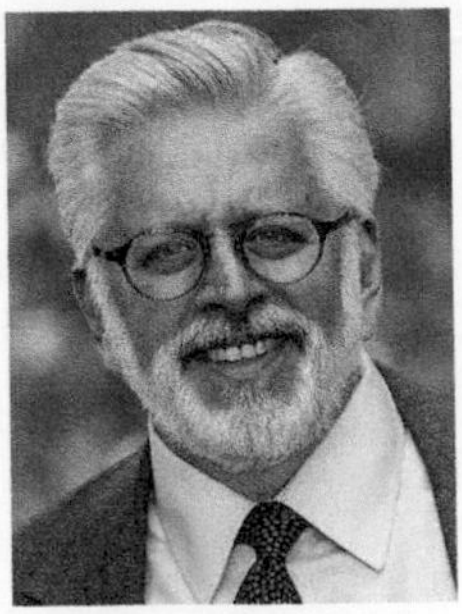

Adam S. Landsman, DPM, PhD, FACFAS
Editor

I had the opportunity to serve as guest editor for *Clinics in Podiatric Medicine and Surgery* in 1996 and again in 2009, for issues that focused on wound care and implantable biologic materials. Since that time, the use of biologic materials in the operating room has flourished. Advancements in the procurement and preparation of allografts and xenografts have helped these materials make their way to the operating room table. In the process, new synthetic materials also became available that resemble natural materials with regard to tissue incorporation, but also improve on various mechanical characteristics.

With respect to this issue, cartilage, bone, and collagen allografts are used in the operating room to reconstruct joints, fuse bones, and repair cartilage. Placental membrane and mesenchymal stem cells are also used to treat tendon and joint pathologies. In Dr Petranto's article, "Multiple Foot and Ankle Applications of the Artelon Implant: Three Case Reports and a Review of the Literature," a series of cases is presented in which a synthetic material can also be used for reconstructive applications. There is also a head-to-head comparison between living skin allografts and a laboratory-formed skin substitute for the treatment of venous leg ulcers. In each of these articles, the ultimate goal is to repair and replace injured tissues.

In the article entitled, "Near Infrared Imaging Spectroscopy for Assessing Skin and Wound Oxygen Perfusion," the use of near infrared spectroscopy is used to assess skin and wound oxygenation and vascular perfusion. I strongly believe that this is a new technology whose time has arrived. The oxygenation, perfusion, and incorporation of a biologic material are the ultimate proof of biocompatibility. In the future, this technology will help us to understand what works in our patients and what does not.

Clin Podiatr Med Surg 35 (2018) xiii–xiv
https://doi.org/10.1016/j.cpm.2018.03.001
0891-8422/18/© 2018 Published by Elsevier Inc.

As a bioengineer, I have been fortunate enough to work with many brilliant scientists who enabled me to pull back the curtain and glimpse into the future of implantable biologics and tissue engineering. As a surgeon, I have spent countless hours in the operating room and have witnessed firsthand the transfer of technology that I believe ultimately improves the lives of our patients. It is my privilege to have the opportunity to share some of these great new ideas with you today.

Adam S. Landsman, DPM, PhD, FACFAS
Division of Podiatric Surgery
Department of Surgery
Cambridge Health Alliance
Harvard Medical School
1493 Cambridge Street, Floor 2
Cambridge, MA 02139, USA

E-mail address:
alandsman@cha.harvard.edu

Complications Following Allograft and Xenograft Resurfacing of the First Metatarsal Head: A Case Series

Jason A. Kayce, DPM[a], Jennifer Buchanan, DPM[b],
Adam S. Landsman, DPM, PhD[c,*]

KEYWORDS

• Joint resurfacing • Allograft • Xenograft • Hallux limitus • Hallux rigidus
• Metatarsal phalangeal joint • Decellularized collagen • Foreign body reaction

KEY POINTS

- In some cases, resurfacing of the metatarsal head with a decellularized collagen material may result in severe erosion and destruction of the underlying bone.
- Foreign body reactions to decellularized collagen may occur.
- Bone destruction following joint resurfacing can be treated with joint replacement if sufficient healthy bone remains.

INTRODUCTION

Hallux limitus/rigidus is the second most common pathologic condition of the first metatarsophalangeal joint. However, surgical treatment options remain somewhat limited.[1] Surgical techniques include both joint salvage and joint destructive procedures. The latter represents joint arthrodesis, total joint replacement, or semijoint resurfacing, whereas the former includes a cheilectomy, decompression osteotomy, or the interpositional arthroplasty.[1]

Original interposition arthroplasties involved placement of an autograft within the joint interface, often leading to donor site morbidity and a less-than-optimal clinical outcome.[1] As a result, recent developments have geared toward placement of a decellularized xenograft or allograft within the joint interface.

Disclosure: The authors have nothing to disclose.
[a] Paradise Valley Foot and Ankle, 4611 E Shea Boulevard #160, Phoenix, AZ 85028, USA; [b] Division of Podiatric Surgery, Cambridge Health Alliance, 1493 Cambridge Street, Cambridge, MA 02139, USA; [c] Division of Podiatric Surgery, Department of Surgery, Cambridge Health Alliance, Harvard Medical School, 1493 Cambridge Street, Floor 2, Cambridge, MA 02139, USA
* Corresponding author.
E-mail address: alandsman@cha.harvard.edu

Clin Podiatr Med Surg 35 (2018) 271–280
https://doi.org/10.1016/j.cpm.2018.02.001
podiatric.theclinics.com

There are numerous collagen bio-scaffold products available with variable surgical applications. When evaluating the application of an interpositional joint collagen graft, some products may serve better than others. The graft must provide strength to withstand the shearing and compressive forces within a weight-bearing joint, without being too bulky to limit joint motion. As the thickness of a graft increases, so does the load capacity; however, the graft loses malleability. There are both cross-linked and non–cross-linked graft products available. The strength of a graft increases proportionally to the amount of cross-linking present. On the other hand, artificial cross-linking decreases the susceptibility of the collagen to undergo enzymatic degradation, thereby limiting incorporation into host tissues.[2,3]

Human or bovine dermal matrix grafts provide an ideal compromise of the aforementioned criteria in comparison with other commercially available products. Porcine small intestine submucosa is thin, weak, highly cross-linked, and, therefore, unable to withstand forces through a weight-bearing joint.[4] Equine pericardium is typically cross-linked, restraining incorporation into host tissue.[4] Bovine and porcine bio-scaffolds are similar to human dermal matrix in strength as well as non–cross-linked availability; however, human tissue may decrease the risk of graft-host rejection.[4] Donated human and bovine dermal matrix can withstand forces within a joint interface and is available non–cross-linked to allow improved incorporation.

In making the decision to resurface a joint, the advantages and disadvantages must be carefully weighed. First and foremost is the condition of the joint before surgery and the reasons why the surgery is necessary. Joint resurfacing is designed to recreate the gliding cartilaginous surface. In cases whereby the preoperative range of motion is poor or is zero, the reason for this must be ascertained and addressed. In some cases, large osteophytes may limit the range of motion; these can be removed, making the process of joint restoration much more simple. However, in other cases, hallux limitus or rigidus is the result of elongated metatarsal, subchondral defects, such as cysts, metatarsal elevation, sesamoid pathology, or extensive damage to the phalangeal base. In these cases, joint replacement or arthrodesis may make more sense.

Another consideration is whether or not inflammatory arthritis, such as rheumatoid arthritis or gout, is present. In these cases, it is more likely that the chronic inflammation will have a destructive effect on the collagen before it can become fully incorporated into the joint surface, because collagen is a competitive inhibitor of matrix metalloproteinases.

At this time, the authors have completed 10 cases in which the first metatarsal head was resurfaced using either a decellularized collagen allograft or xenograft. The technique used to perform the joint resurfacing has been previously described.[5] In 3 of these cases, significant degeneration and erosion of the metatarsal head became apparent approximately 6 to 9 months postoperatively. In all 3 cases, the salvage for this was to remove the remnants of the graft as well as resect degenerative bone and cartilage. The damaged joint was then repaired in 2 of the cases, as described here, using a silicone joint. In the third case where boney erosion of the first metatarsal head occurred, a metallic hemi implant was used instead. Although this patient recovered without complications, there were some technical complications unrelated to her joint pathology that made her particular case unsuitable to be included as part of this series.

CASE REPORT 1

An active, 48-year-old Caucasian woman with no significant past medical history presented to the clinic, under the care of the authors, with a chief complaint of pain in her right first metatarsophalangeal joint. She reported no history of trauma to the area. Her symptoms were most notable with walking and running and had been increasingly debilitating for several months. Treatment to date consisted of supportive shoe gear, over-the-counter nonsteroidal antiinflammatory medications, and rest before being seen in our clinic. She reported minimal relief.

On physical examination, pain was elicited with direct palpation and manipulation of the right first metatarsophalangeal joint. Range of motion was painful and limited to the right first metatarsophalangeal joint. The patient had palpable pedal pulses, and sensation was grossly intact to light touch. Initial radiographic analysis displayed mild elevatus of the first metatarsal and increased length of the first metatarsal. There was no significant joint space narrowing, yet subchondral sclerosis could be appreciated to the base of the proximal phalanx. Images revealed central subchondral cystic formation within the central aspect of the first metatarsal head. The patient was treated conservatively with shoe gear modification, activity modification, over-the-counter nonsteroidal antiinflammatory medications, and rest. The patient returned to the clinic several months later, reporting no improvement of her symptoms. At this time, she reported exhaustion with conservative care and interest in surgical intervention.

Initial surgical intervention consisted of a cheilectomy and interpositional arthroplasty with collagen allograft to the first metatarsophalangeal joint. In standard fashion, a dorsomedial incision was created over the first metatarsophalangeal joint. The incision was deepened through skin and subcutaneous tissue with care taken to avoid pertinent neurovascular structures. A linear capsular incision was then created medial and parallel to the extensor hallucis longus tendon. The capsule and periosteal tissues were then reflected to reveal the head of the first metatarsal and base of the proximal phalanx. Dorsal, medial, and lateral exostoses were appreciated to the head of the first metatarsal and base of the proximal phalanx, which were subsequently reduced without incident. Evaluation of the articular surfaces revealed an erosion encompassing approximately 40% of the first metatarsal head, which was subchondrally drilled in a microfracture technique using a 0.045-in smooth Kirschner wire.

Following removal of osteophytes, joint motion was greatly improved; it was decided to proceed with the application of a non–cross-linked, acellular dermal matrix composed of donated human tissue to the first metatarsal (Dermacell, LifeNet Health, Virginia Beach, VA, USA). The authors performed a unique standard surgical technique when performing an interpositional arthroplasty of the first metatarsophalangeal joint, as shown in **Fig. 1**. The allograft is folded in half and stitched along one side with an absorbable suture. The collagen sleeve is then passed over the first metatarsal head. Care is taken to maintain a taut collagenous surface to minimize wrinkles within the joint. The material is firmly sutured along the medial aspect with an absorbable suture and is captured into the capsule during closure to prevent implant migration.[5]

The patient's immediate postoperative course was uneventful. She was placed in a surgical shoe and allowed to bear weight as tolerated immediately postoperatively. Her clinical appearance displayed progression of healing as expected without complication. She was transitioned to athletic, supportive shoe gear and allowed to bear weight as tolerated 1 week postoperatively. She was allowed more demanding physical activity at 4 weeks. Serial radiographs were obtained immediately postoperatively, 4 weeks, and 8 weeks postoperatively. No surgical complications were apparent, and she seemed to be healing within normal limits.

Approximately 10 months after surgery, the patient returned to the clinic complaining of pain and swelling to the associated joint. Radiographs displayed significant

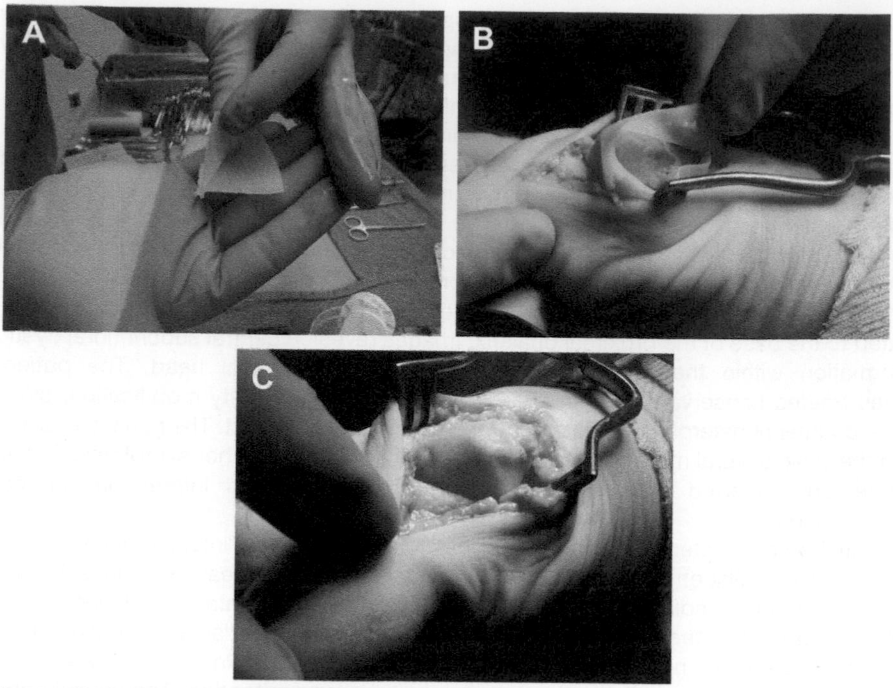

Fig. 1. These intraoperative photographs illustrate the surgical technique of an interpositional arthroplasty of the first metatarsal phalangeal joint. (*A*) An acellular, non–cross-linked, human dermal matrix allograft is folded in half and stitched along one side with an absorbable suture. (*B*) The collagen sleeve is then passed over the first metatarsal head. Care is taken to maintain the tautness of the collagen as it is stretched across the metatarsal head, so that no wrinkles occur within the joint. (*C*) The material is firmly sutured along the medial aspect with an absorbable suture. Note the way that the collagen contours to the shape of the metatarsal head. The graft is captured along with the capsule and periosteum during closure to prevent it from migrating.

progression of erosive changes within the first metatarsal head as well as the proximal phalangeal base of the hallux. An exhaustive list of differential diagnoses was formulated. Objective data indicated that surgical exploration was necessary at this time. Subsequent surgical intervention would consist of intraoperative evaluation of the first metatarsophalangeal joint, bone resection, cultures, Gram stain, and total joint replacement with a silicone total joint and grommets.

The patient returned to the operating room, where the same dorsomedial incision was carried over the first metatarsophalangeal joint. Dissection was deepened to the level of the joint capsule. No purulence, malodor, discoloration, or other signs of infection were appreciated. A dorsomedial capsular incision was created medial and parallel to the extensor hallucis longus tendon. The capsule appeared quite hypertrophied but revealed no other signs of infection. No bleeding or synovitis was appreciated within the joint.

On exposure of the first metatarsal head, quite extensive erosive changes were appreciated to nearly 70% of the articular surface, as displayed in **Fig. 2**. Wound cultures were obtained. The metatarsal head was resected and sent for microbiologic and pathologic evaluation. The remaining distal aspect of the metatarsal displayed numerous cystic lesions, which was packed with calcium sulfate and calcium

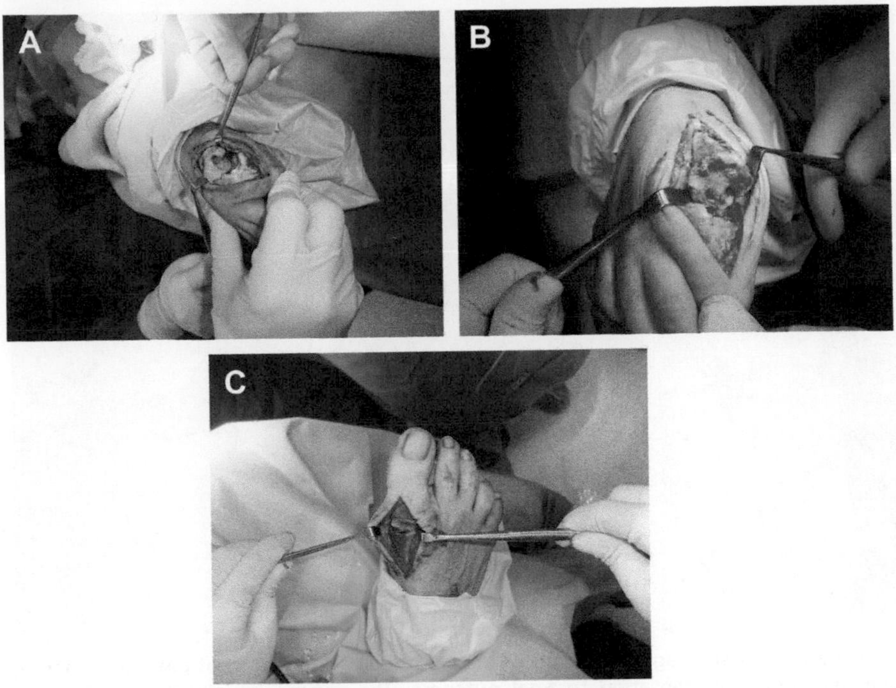

Fig. 2. These images demonstrate the intraoperative findings in case 1, approximately 10 months after placement of an acellular, non–cross-linked human dermal matrix, which was used as an interpositional joint graft. Significant erosive changes encompass nearly 75% of the first metatarsal head (*A*). The eroded first metatarsal head was resected and sent to pathology for analysis. Several cysts were encountered at this time (*B*). Because of the size of the remaining defect, additional bone resection was required to reach a stable foundation for total joint implantation. A silicone first metatarsal phalangeal joint implant with grommets was seated into the joint (*C*).

phosphate substrate (Pro-Dense, Wright Medical Technology, Memphis, TN, USA) in preparation for placement of a total joint silicone insert with grommets. No obvious degeneration was observed on the base of the first proximal phalanx.

After preparing the calcium phosphate substrate and allotting the proper set time, the metatarsal still did not seem sufficient to withstand the loading capacity of a total silicone implant. Because of the patient's increased first metatarsal length, there was adequate bone available to allow for resection of an additional 5-mm portion of the distal metatarsal, which ultimately exposed sufficient bone stock to secure an implant.

According to standard manufactured protocol, both the metatarsal shaft and the base of the proximal phalanx were prepared for acceptance of a total joint implant. A size 1S silicone total joint implant with grommets (Wright Medical) was seated within the first metatarsal phalangeal joint. The surgical site was thoroughly irrigated. The hypertrophied capsule was reduced to a healthy layer of capsular tissue, which was followed by closure of the capsule, subcutaneous tissue, and skin. The patient was placed in a posterior splint with crutches and ordered non–weight bearing to the extremity, secondary to the fragile nature of the bony structure due to cystic progression. Preoperative and postoperative radiographs show the degenerated metatarsal and subsequent repair (**Fig. 3**).

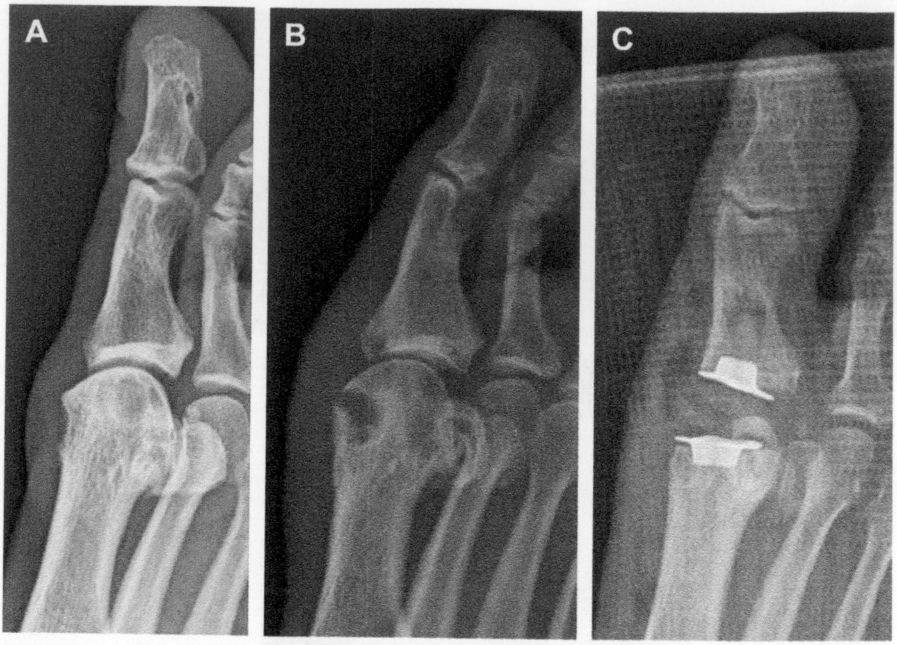

Fig. 3. Each of these images represents a medial oblique radiograph of patient 1, ranging from her original presentation to final outcome. The patient initially displayed clinical and radiographic symptoms consistent with hallux limitus. In addition, there were subchondral degenerative changes (*A*). The patient underwent a cheilectomy and interpositional arthroplasty of the first metatarsal phalangeal joint with placement of an acellular, non–cross-linked collagen allograft. Approximately 10 months postoperatively, radiographic analysis revealed acceleration of subchondral degenerative changes and significant progression of cystic formation within the first metatarsal head and possibly in the base of the proximal phalanx (*B*). After surgical exploration and bone resection, a total joint replacement was performed with placement of a silicone first metatarsal phalangeal total joint with grommets (*C*).

Postoperatively, both Gram stain and culture revealed no growth of organisms. Bone pathology, however, did reveal irregular lamellar bone and marrow with degenerative changes and necrosis. Peripheral tissues displayed a focus of acute inflammation, granulation tissue, fibrosis, and bone resorption, as depicted in **Fig. 4**. Numerous multinucleated giant cells were appreciated. When visualized under a polarizing microscope, a focal foreign body giant cell encapsulates polarizable foreign material. These data revealed evidence of an encapsulation reaction to foreign material, thought to be the collagen allograft.

The patient was followed in the clinic 1 week, 2 weeks, 4 weeks, and 10 weeks postoperatively. She was dispensed a fixed ankle walking boot 1 week postoperatively, at which time she could begin transition to protected weight-bearing status. She progressed to an athletic sneaker at 2 weeks and began physical therapy at 4 weeks. Serial radiographs were obtained throughout her postoperative course, which revealed maintenance of the grommets within the first metatarsal and proximal phalanx. There was no further progression of destruction within the first metatarsophalangeal joint. She was allowed full return to athletic activity 10 weeks postoperatively, at which time she was discharged and allowed to return to the clinic as needed. She was

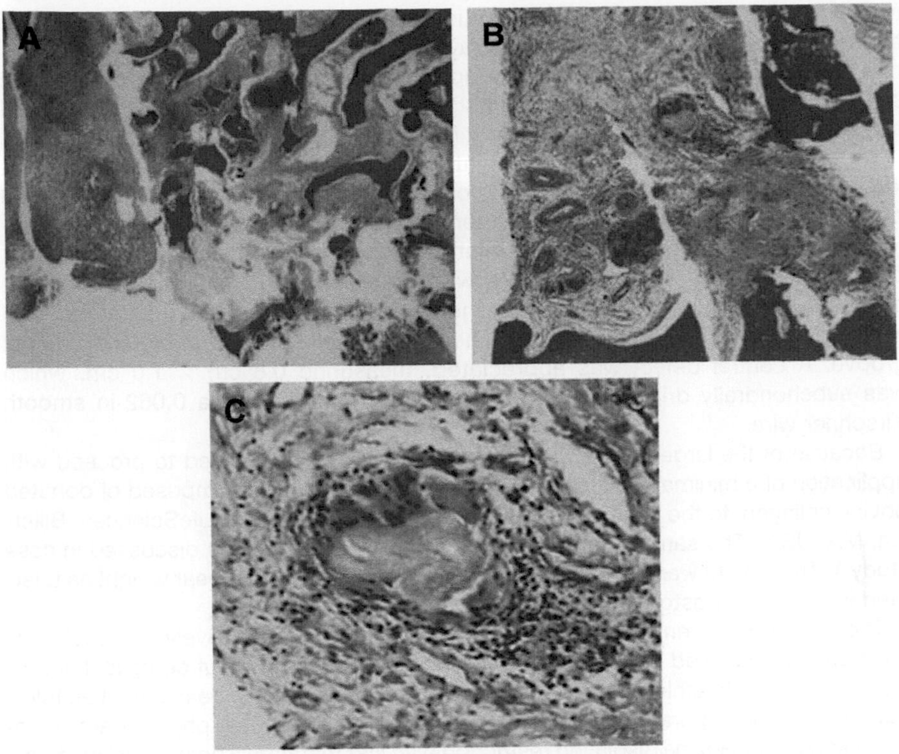

Fig. 4. The images demonstrate histologic evaluation of the first metatarsal head approximately 10 months after placement of an acellular, non–cross-linked allograft. Irregular interrupted lamellar bone and marrow with degenerative changes and necrosis is visualized (*A*). The peripheral tissue displays a focus of acute inflammation, granulation tissue, fibrosis, and bone resorption (*A*, hematoxylin-eosin [H&E]). Numerous multinucleated giant cells are representative of a foreign body reaction (*B*, H&E). When visualized under polarizing microscope, a focal foreign body giant cell encapsulates polarizable foreign material (*C*, H&E).

seen again 1 year postoperatively with full activity and good range of motion at the first metatarsal phalangeal joint and without any concerns of pain.

CASE REPORT 2

An active 44-year-old Caucasian man with no significant past medical history presented to the clinic with a chief complaint of pain to bilateral first metatarsal phalangeal joints. He denied any history of trauma to the areas and reported pain for many years. He reported pain to left as more severe than the contralateral joint. He had previously seen another physician who dispensed custom orthotics and recommended supportive shoe gear, over-the-counter nonsteroidal antiinflammatory medications, and rest. The patient reported exhaustion with conservative measures and interest in surgical intervention.

On physical examination, significant limitation of dorsiflexion was appreciated at the first metatarsal phalangeal joint bilaterally. Pain was elicited with end range of motion, more notably to the left first metatarsal phalangeal joint. The patient had palpable +2 pedal pulses, and sensation was grossly intact to light touch. Initial radiographic analysis displayed elevation of the first metatarsal and increased length of the first metatarsal. Moderate metatarsus adductus could be appreciated. The first metatarsal head and proximal phalangeal base displayed osteophyte formation. Moderate asymmetric joint space narrowing could be appreciated, most notably with medial joint space narrowing. Images revealed subchondral cystic formation within the central and lateral aspects of the first metatarsal head.

As with case study 1, initial surgical intervention consisted of a cheilectomy and interpositional arthroplasty but with collagen xenograft to the first metatarsal phalangeal joint. The same incision approach and dissection technique was performed to reveal the head of the first metatarsal and base of the proximal phalanx. Dorsal, medial, and lateral exostoses were appreciated to the head of the first metatarsal and base of the proximal phalanx, which were subsequently reduced without incident. The first metatarsal head revealed erosions along the sagittal groove. A central defect was appreciated, measuring 0.8 cm × 1.0 cm, which was subchondrally drilled in a microfracture technique using a 0.062-in smooth Kirschner wire.

Because of the large central cartilaginous defect, it was decided to proceed with application of a minimally cross-linked acellular dermal matrix composed of donated bovine collagen, to the first metatarsal head (SurgiMend, Integra LifeSciences, Billerica, MA, USA). The same application technique was used as was discussed in case study 1. The patient was placed in a surgical shoe and allowed to bear weight as tolerated immediately postoperatively.

The patient was seen 1 week, 4 weeks, and 7 weeks postoperatively. His postoperative course displayed progression of healing as expected without complication. He was transitioned to athletic, supportive shoe gear and allowed to bear weight as tolerated 1 week postoperatively. He was allowed more demanding physical activity at 4 weeks. At 7 weeks, he displayed restriction with first metatarsal phalangeal joint dorsiflexion and was fitted and dispensed a Dynasplint to assist with gaining proper range of motion to the joint.

Serial radiographs were obtained immediately postoperatively to reveal maintenance of proper joint alignment. Images at 7 weeks display maintenance of the joint space along with cystic changes within the first metatarsal, as seen previously. Four months after undergoing a left first metatarsophalangeal joint interpositional arthroplasty, the patient returned to the clinic complaining of continued joint stiffness but no pain. Radiographs displayed significant progression of erosive changes within the first metatarsal head.

As with case study 1, a similar list of differential diagnoses was formulated and treatment measures were discussed. The patient returned to the operating room, where the same dorsomedial incision was carried over the first metatarsal phalangeal joint. Dissection was deepened to the level of the joint capsule. No purulence, malodor, discoloration, or other signs of infection were appreciated; but significant scar tissue was encountered. A dorsomedial capsular incision was created medial and parallel to the extensor hallucis longus tendon. The capsule displayed no signs of infection. On exposure of the first metatarsal head, quite extensive erosive changes were appreciated centrally within the first metatarsal head to the level of the crista plantarly. Unlike case study 1, a plug of soft tissue consistent with the original xenograft was visualized within the cyst. This material was removed and sent to pathology and microbiology for evaluation. A sagittal saw was used to resect the head of the first metatarsal and base of the proximal phalanx in preparation for placement of a total joint implant. No further cysts were encountered after resection of the first metatarsal head. The remainder of the procedure proceeded as discussed in case study 1, with placement of a silicone (Silastic, Dow Corning, Midland, MI, USA) total joint implant with grommets (Wright

Medical, size 2S). The patient was placed in a surgical shoe with crutches and ordered non–weight bearing to the extremity.

The pathology report eventually returned to display findings consistent with those in case study 1. The tissue flap within the cyst of the first metatarsal displayed a cellular response consistent with a foreign body giant cell reaction. The head of the first metatarsal and base of the proximal phalanx displayed chronic inflammatory cell infiltrate with fat necrosis, fibrosis, and, once again, foreign body giant cell reaction.

The patient was followed in the clinic 1 week, 3 weeks, and 14 weeks postoperatively. He was allowed to transition to protected weight-bearing status in a surgical shoe at 1 week postoperatively. He progressed to an athletic sneaker at 2 weeks and began physical therapy at 3 weeks. Serial radiographs were obtained throughout his postoperative course, which revealed maintenance of the grommets within the first metatarsal and proximal phalanx. There was no further progression of destruction with the first metatarsal phalangeal joint. He returned to the clinic 14 weeks postoperatively, at which time he was discharged and allowed to return to the clinic as needed.

DISCUSSION

Approximately 1 in 40 individuals older than 50 years of age have osteoarthritis of the first metatarsal phalangeal joint. Various surgical and nonsurgical options have been offered to patients but none with constant, reproducible, positive outcomes. More recently, resurfacing the first metatarsal head with autograft or allograft collagen product has been entertained in an attempt to provide pain relief while maintaining anatomic structures and, thus, biomechanical parameters within the lower extremity. An initial case report using Graftjacket (Wright Medical) (acellular human derma bioscaffold) resurfacing of the metatarsal head with adjunctive hemi-implant in the proximal phalanx resulted in less pain and improved function during the postoperative course, whereas a biopsy of the joint demonstrated neo-cartilage formation.[6] A 5-year follow-up of 6 patients using Graftjacket interpositional grafting showed an increase in the AOFAS score from 38.0 to 65.8, and all patients were satisfied with their surgical outcome.[1,7] Although studies are limited at this time, especially long term clinical follow-up, these results suggest there is a place for joint resurfacing for the management of hallux limitus/rigidus.

Surgical treatment of hallux limitus/rigidus in active patients remains limited. In this case, a joint salvage procedure was first attempted with placement of an acellular, non–cross-linked collagen allograft. Postoperatively, it became evident that this patient developed an encapsulation reaction to foreign material, leading to an accelerated progression of degenerative changes within the first metatarsal phalangeal joint. Revision surgery involved placement of a silicone total joint implant, which the patient healed uneventfully.

To date, there is no published literature presenting such a complication with the application of an acellular, non–cross-linked human dermal matrix. It is hypothesized that relative contraindications to the interpositional arthroplasty with an allograft may include the presence of preoperative subchondral cysts and/or an increase in first metatarsal length. Increased metatarsal length may result in jamming of the joint secondary to functional hallux limitus. Until further studies are developed to investigate these hypotheses, it is recommended to decompress the joint via osteotomy and to remove the entire wall of any cysts before placement of an interpositional allograft or xenograft.

In the authors' experience, salvage procedures are largely dictated by the quantity and quality of bone remaining after removal of damaged bone. In this case series, one salvage option using a silicone total joint with grommets was shown. The authors have also performed a salvage with a metallic hemi implant, which resulted in excessive shortening of the first metatarsal and transfer lesions to the area beneath the second metatarsal. In cases such as this, whereby resection of damaged bone is extensive, fusion, possibly with bone graft to restore length, may prove to be the most reliable option for salvage.

REFERENCES

1. Berlet GC, Hyer CF, Lee TH, et al. Interpositional arthroplasty of the first MTP joint using a regenerative tissue matrix for the treatment of advanced hallux rigidus. Foot Ankle Int 2008;29(1):10–21.
2. Charulatha V, Rajaram A. Influence of different crosslinking treatments on the physical properties of collagen membranes. Biomaterials 2003;24(5):759–67.
3. Weadock KS, Miller EJ, Keuffel EL, et al. Effect of physical crosslinking methods on collagen-fiber durability in proteolytic solutions. J Biomed Mater Res 1996;32(2): 221–6.
4. Cornwell KG, Landsman A, James KS. Extracellular matrix biomaterials for soft tissue repair. Clin Podiatr Med Surg 2009;26(4):507–23.
5. Landsman AS [Chapter 3]. In: Southerland J, Boberg JS, Downey MS, et al, editors. McGlamry's comprehensive textbook of foot and ankle surgery, 2 vol. Set. Wolters-Kluwer Pub; 2013. p. 24–36.
6. Brigido SA, Troiano M, Schoenhaus H. Biologic resurfacing of the ankle and first metatarsophalangeal joint: case studies with a 2-year follow-up. Clin Podiatr Med Surg 2009;26(4):633–45.
7. Hyer CF, Granata JD, Berlet GC, et al. Interpositional arthroplasty of the first metatarsophalangeal joint using a regenerative tissue matrix for the treatment of advanced hallux rigidus: 5-year case series follow-up. Foot Ankle Spec 2012; 5(4):249–52.

Allograft Cartilage Replacements

Michael H. Theodoulou, DPM[a], Laura Bohman, DPM, AACFAS[b,*]

KEYWORDS

• Allograft • Scaffold • Cartilage • Talus • Foot

KEY POINTS

- Articular cartilage is a complex structure of cellular chondrocytes and extracellular matrix that provides frictionless movement and resists compressive forces; however, it lacks the ability to restore itself after damage.
- Allograft tissues are used with increasing frequency to help restore native cartilage, eliminate donor site morbidity, and, most frequently, provide a single stage surgery.
- Acellular allograft scaffolds can include products using components of extracellular matrix and serve as a skeleton to promote the creation of hyaline-like cartilage.
- Cellular allografts provide viable chondrocyte cells to promote healing. Often juvenile samples that demonstrate greater cellular density and increased mitotic activity among other capabilities are used.
- Allograft tissues are often used in foot and ankle surgery for repair of articular cartilage damage.

INTRODUCTION

The body's ability to repair injured articular cartilage is poor due to the inherent physiology of cartilage. Joint arthritis, whether through injury or increasing age, is a prevalent condition. Treatment of an articular cartilage injury may include arthroplasty, fusion, or repair. A popular pathway of treatment in a salvageable joint is often to avoid donor site morbidity and place increased effort to re-establish native cartilage with the use of allografts. This article discusses current research on acellular and cellular allografts for articular cartilage restoration.

Disclosure: Dr M.H. Theodoulou is a paid consultant for Arthrex and Cartiva surgical device companies, and BSN medical. All other authors declare that they have no conflicts of interest.

[a] Department of Surgery, Cambridge Health Alliance, Harvard Medical School, 1493 Cambridge Street, Cambridge, MA 02139, USA; [b] Podiatry Associates of Cincinnati, 10615 Montgomery Road, Suite 100, Cincinnati, OH 45242, USA
* Corresponding author.
E-mail address: bohman.laura@gmail.com

Clin Podiatr Med Surg 35 (2018) 281–293
https://doi.org/10.1016/j.cpm.2018.02.003

ARTICULAR CARTILAGE ANATOMY

Articular cartilage is a combination of relatively few cells, chondrocytes, and extracellular matrix. It lacks blood vessels, lymphatic drainage, and innervation, and it receives nutrients via synovial joint fluid. Articular cartilage along with synovial fluid allows for smooth gliding of the joint and a functional joint that can adapt to and resist compressive forces.[1] Articular cartilage is arranged in 4 layers of differing composition and organization of chondrocytes and extracellular matrix. These layers provide adherence of the cartilage to bone, channels for nutrient dispersal, collagen framework to house necessary macromolecules, and a smooth frictionless surface for joint motion. These layers in composition and thickness are specialized for different joints, such as the knee versus the ankle (**Fig. 1**). In general, chondrocytes are the cellular component of cartilage that creates and organizes the extracellular matrix. The extracellular matrix is composed of fluid, collagen, proteoglycans, and small amounts of other proteins. Collagen forms the skeleton of the cartilage housing chondrocytes, fluid, and proteoglycans. Proteoglycans are molecules that expand in fluid to provide resistance against compression.[1] Overall, the complex network, elasticity, and lack of capability of self-repair of cartilage provides insight to the difficulty in attempted restoration.

HISTORY OF CARTILAGE REPAIR

Throughout history it was widely known that cartilage lacked the ability to heal or restore itself after significant damage, but it was not until the late 1950s that the physiology of cartilage nutrition and repair was described.[2,3] In 1959, subchondral drilling was described by Insall and colleagues,[3,4] as a way to repair articular cartilage injury using the subchondral bone as a vascular supply to stimulate healing. The most current technique of microfracture, that is still in use today was described by Steadman and colleagues.[3,5] In 1976, Gross and colleagues[6] used osteochondral allografts for repair after tumor resections in the knee, and in the mid-1980s, Yamashita and colleagues[3,7] used osteochondral autografts to treat

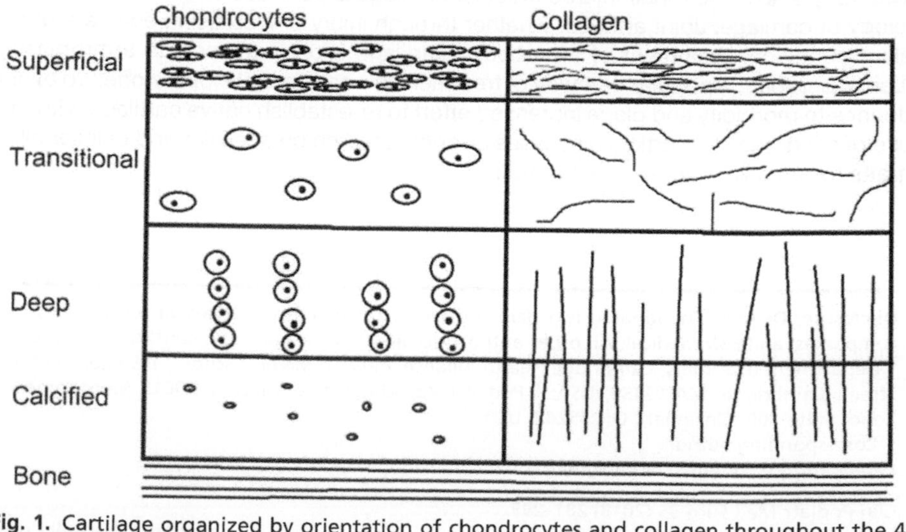

Fig. 1. Cartilage organized by orientation of chondrocytes and collagen throughout the 4 differentiated layers.

osteochondritis dissecans. Further research to decrease donor site morbidity, prevent incongruences with transplantations, and allow for more readily available graft has led us to more recent advances in articular cartilage restoration using allograft tissues.

TYPES OF ALLOGRAFT

Allograft cartilage replacements may consist of both cellular and acellular products. Acellular products include scaffolds and allograft tissues that possess extracellular matrix, proteins, and growth factors capable of producing chondro-conductive, chondro-inductive, and chondrogenic influence to the native tissue. Cellular products include fresh frozen grafts and cryopreserved juvenile cartilage that can be presented as particulate or whole grafts.

Acellular

Historically, scaffolds have been divided into synthetic versus naturally derived materials. Clearly, the challenge has always been associated with implant–post integration. Synthetic materials frequently are hydrogel and electrospun fibers. The advantage of these scaffolds include controlled degradation, high reproducibility, high mechanical strength, and easy manipulation of product. The negative of this type of scaffold includes failure to have presence of cell recognition signals. Natural scaffolds include polymers of agarose, alginate, chitosan, and hyaluronate. There are protein scaffolds to include collagen, gelatin, fibrin, and silk. Advantages of natural scaffolds include biocompatibility but, unfortunately, these have poor mechanical strength and higher degradation rates. Recently, hybrid scaffolds have been of interest because they provide potential for high stiffness properties, tension, and compression while exhibiting the viscoelastic response seen in hydrogels and native cartilage tissue. Fibers to include combinations of hyaluronic acid and hydrogel with varying pore sizes have been evaluated. Of interest is whether these hybrids demonstrate improved differentiated chondrocytes as well as improved expression of extracellular matrix, proteins, type I and type II collagen, and aggrecan compared with synthetics. As discussed previously, one of the benefits for synthetic scaffolds is their ability to control degradation. This also leads to some concern regarding degradative byproduct and its potential detrimental effects. Lam and colleagues[8] studied polycaprolactone (PCL) as a biomaterial. They looked at both the synthetic and composites through both in vitro and in vivo study. Both samples demonstrated no molecular weight changes after 6 months and a maximum loss of 7% was found in the composite scaffold in vivo. There was an appreciated slight increase in crystallinity. Histologic examination of the in vivo samples did demonstrate good biocompatibility with no adverse host tissue reactions at 6 months.

Mintz and Cooper[9] appreciated that these hybrids did encourage a more rounded chondrocyte morphology without detriment to proliferation viability. They also found that this hybrid expressed mechanical properties similar to that of native cartilage in both tension and compression, and it was able to maintain seating chondrocyte phenotype.[9]

Oliveira and colleagues[10] looked at cornstarch PCL scaffolds in combination with bovine articular chondrocytes. After these were cultured for 6 weeks, they used scanning electron microscopy and varying stains to include different assays and immunolocalization for collagen types 1 and 2. They confirmed that the scaffolds demonstrated chondrocytes of normal morphologic features with extensive cell differentiation.

Unfortunately, on systematic review by Shimozono and colleagues,[11] there are few clinical studies with appropriate level of evidence and good methodological quality when evaluating scaffold therapy and management of osteochondral lesions of the talus. Most studies demonstrated scaffolds consisting of autologous chondrocyte implantation or other autologous biologic, such as bone marrow aspirate or platelet rich plasma. Christensen and colleagues[12] demonstrated poor osteochondral repair in the knee using a biomimetic collagen scaffold.

Acellular allograft scaffolds can include products using components of extracellular matrix, proteins, and collagen. This type of product serves as a scaffold allowing for creation of hyaline-like cartilage. It may favorably have reduced cost compared with some of the cellular allografts. Currently available is a dehydrated, micronized allogeneic cartilage that can be combined with autograft products, such as bone marrow aspirate, full blood, or platelet-rich plasma to enhance healing articular injury. Again there is no cellular component to this product, but it does possess identified type II collagen as well as proteoglycans and cartilaginous growth factors to prompt a chondral conductive and inductive process. The chondrogenic aspect of this product is based on bone marrow stimulation with the microfracture of the lesion.

There are few clinical studies both in vitro and in vivo using extracellular matrix cartilage allograft. Desa[13] reported on 9 patients where this was performed on the talus with an average lesion size of approximately 132 mm^2. End-time outcome was 12 months. They reported on 7 excellent and 2 good outcomes.[13]

Cellular

In an effort to enhance healing of articular injury, there has now been utilization of particulate cartilage allograft. This does possess viable cells. Donors are usually less than 3 years of age but can be up to 13 years old. The juvenile cartilage is found to have higher concentration of chondrocytes. In a study by Liu and colleagues,[14] comparing samples of juvenile bovine cartilage and adult cartilage, they identified that juvenile samples demonstrated greater cellular density, increased mitotic activity, elevated glycosaminoglycan, and enhanced activity of matrix metallopeptidase 2 activity. In vitro examination of the both adult and juvenile cartilage during 4 weeks culture incubation demonstrated only juvenile cartilage was capable of generating new cartilage with increased proteoglycan and type II collagen with no type I evident. Furthermore, genetic expression for cartilage growth and expansion was found up-regulated in juvenile cartilage whereas up-regulation for genes crucial in structural integrity was appreciated in adult cartilage. Unfortunately, there remains little research confirming persistence of type II collagen without dedifferentiation back to type I.

In a study by Vira and colleagues,[15] they attempted to use MRI to quantify and compare T2 values, an identified marker of collagen architecture, of native tibiotalar cartilage and those patients repaired with a juvenile particulate allograft for lesions of the talus using a 7T unit. They looked at 7 patients who underwent repair comparing the surrounding normal tissue with the repaired. The average interval following surgery to MRI was 14.9 months. They appreciated higher T2 relaxation times in the repaired cartilage. Increased T2 values do correspond with altered collagen architecture. In patients with osteoarthritis, this suggests early collagen disorganization and altered water content. In acutely repaired tissue with juvenile allograft, it is uncertain what this represents. It is hypothesized that this demonstrates cellular activity with production of collagen and extracellular matrix. The study did not correlate MRI findings with clinical outcomes.

There remain few of studies looking at juvenile particulate cartilage. Saltzman and colleagues,[16] recently published a systematic review of this technique and a retrospective single-center cohort study on their own patients when managing lesions of the talus. The systematic review included 4 studies with a sample of 33 ankles and weighted mean follow-up of 14.3 months. Only 1 ankle was found to require revision as an open procedure with osteochondral allograft at 16 months post–index procedure. Six required nonrevision type procedures at an average of 15 months postoperative. In their own population, 6 patients with mean a follow-up of 13 months reported subjective improvement in pain and motion. Postoperative MRI did confirm continued subchondral edema but no reoperations were performed. In a case series of 9 patients, Van Dyke and colleagues,[17] looked at use of particulated juvenile cartilage in the management of osteochondral defects of the first metatarsal head. With an average follow-up of 3.3 years, 7 of 9 patients reported no pain with recreational activity nor did they require further surgery.

Osteochondral allograft transplantation is frequently used for larger lesions. This is a single-stage procedure that delivers viable articular cartilage and the bone. The challenge is access to graft and preserving chondrocyte viability. Fresh allografts have been preferred to both fresh frozen and cryopreserved with demonstrable ability to maintain improved chondrocyte viability of the donor tissue. It has been shown, however, that chondrocyte viability begins to wane after 28 days postmortem. As a result, it is recommended that fresh allograft be used within 15 days and 28 days postmortem both for safety purposes and for efficacy of the product. The method of cryopreservation varies per manufacturer with each suggesting improved methods to preserve chondrocyte viability. Most methods incorporate tissue culture medium, cytoprotectant solution with varying percentage of DMSO, and controlled freezing with storage below −100°C. Cryopreservation is used to reduce risk of infection transmission, improve storage means, and produce greater ease of access. In a study by Csonge and colleagues,[18] they appreciated that cartilage samples stored in tissue culture medium for 60 days at 4° C demonstrated significantly higher chondrocyte viability when thawed compared with fresh talar cartilage, which was cryopreserved. Current studies identifying chondrocyte viability after cryopreservation suggest typical viability in the low seventies percent at time of thawing with shelf lives up to 2 years.

In review of the literature over the past 15 years regarding fresh talar allografts, most studies demonstrate small sample sizes with the largest being 38 subjects identified in a study by El-Rahidy and colleagues.[19] They appreciated that this was an effective treatment with improved able FAS course and decreased VAS with postoperative MRIs documenting minimal graft subsidence and maintenance of articular congruence in 15 patients. They identified 4 subjects with graft failure.

Hahn and colleagues[20] presented a case series of 13 patients with an average follow-up of 48 months. The average age was 30. Using a FOS ankle hindfoot questionnaire, they determined statistically significant improvement in postoperative pain and activity abilities. They concluded that this was a reasonable procedure for younger adult patients with focal osteochondral talar defects that cannot be addressed with débridement and microfracture. Most recently in 2016, Orr and colleagues,[21] with a sample size of 8 subjects, demonstrated modest improvement in short-term functional outcome scores.

Cryopreserved 3-D meshed grafts are gaining in popularity for focal full thickness lesions in an effort to augment traditional approaches. Recent cartilage restorative techniques studies have been limited to a few surgical technique papers and isolated case studies. Tan and colleagues[22] published on surgical technique for application of this graft to the talus.

Allograft replacements do have notable benefits compared with autologous cartilage grafts. They reduce morbidity associated with donor site, most frequently require a single-stage approach, and, with improved preservation technique, may have easier access to use with greater shelf life. Unfortunately, the tissue is not native to the host and question of postimplant integration remains a concern as well as the cost, without notable intermediate and long-term studies that suggest their efficacy.

CASE PRESENTATIONS

Case 1

A 26-year-old woman presented to an emergency department 20 minutes after traumatic fall while rock climbing. She fell approximately 10 feet on to her left lower extremity. She denied striking her head or loss of consciousness. Her pain remained focused to the left ankle. Radiographs taken in the emergency room confirmed what seemed a partially detached osteochondral fracture of the lateral talar dome (**Fig. 2**). Subsequently an MRI was performed anticipating confirmation of presence of the chondral fracture with anticipation to recommend arthroscopy surgical excision of lesion and débridement of defect. MRI did not suggest chondral fracture with only subchondral contusion, and this was confirmed with musculoskeletal radiologist (**Figs. 3** and **4**). Patient was treated conservatively with immobilization boot and physical medicine. The patient continued to complain of pain in ankle 4 months postinjury despite conservative management. She was provided diagnostic and therapeutic intra-articular corticosteroid injection with dexamethasone phosphate. The patient noted acute relief of symptoms but with relapse of pain 2 weeks post-injection. Advancing her treatment, recommendation for arthroscopic evaluation of the ankle was made with surgery as indicated. Intraoperative findings did confirm osteochondral fracture (**Figs. 5** and **6**) not appreciated on MRI. Surgery

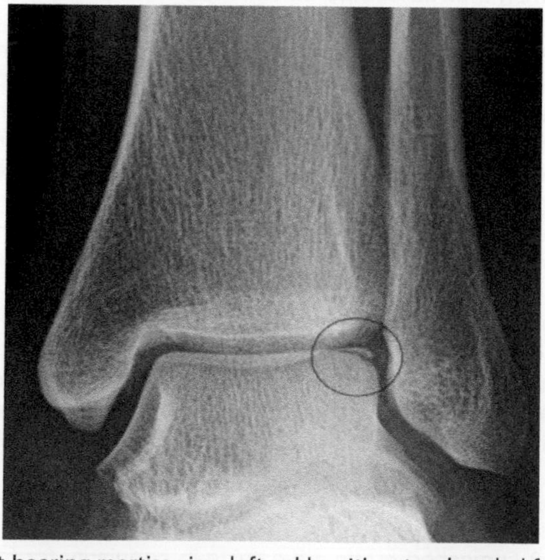

Fig. 2. Non–weight-bearing mortise view left ankle with osteochondral fracture as depicted in the marked circle.

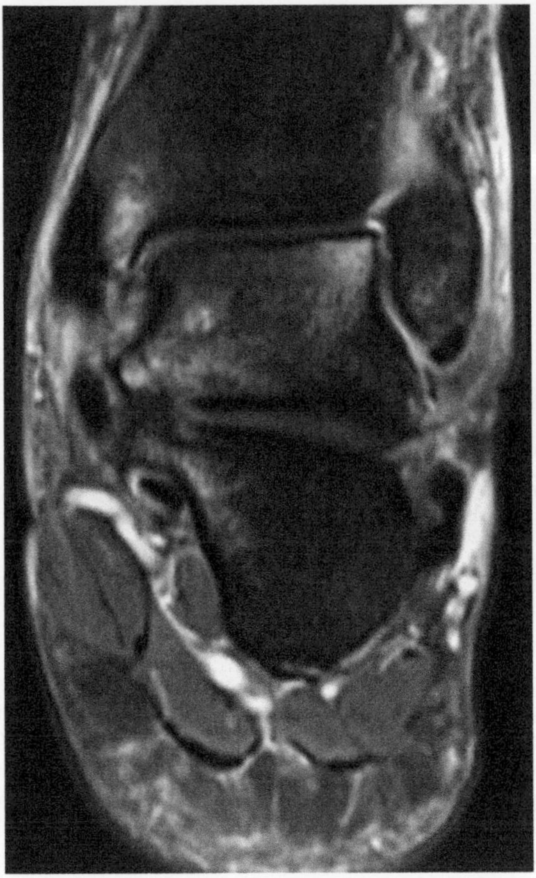

Fig. 3. Coronal MRI T2 image of subchondral contusion.

consisted of excision of the fragment, débridement, microfracture, and application of acellular micronized cartilage matrix secured with fibrin glue (**Fig. 7**). Six-month follow-up with this patient demonstrated asymptomatic ankle and return to all activities.

Case 2

A 60-year-old woman presented with 2-year history of persistent right ankle pain after inversion type injury. She was referred from outside institution having failed conservative management. Initial imaging did confirm osteochondral injury of the medial talar dome with subchondral cystic degeneration. Open arthrotomy and repair of osteochondral defect was recommended, with insertion of a demineralized bone graft for the cyst along with application of cryopreserved mesh cartilage (**Fig. 8**).

Eleven months post-procedure, a follow-up CT scan was performed. Resorption of bone graft was appreciated with persistent small cystic changes, but clinically the patient was asymptomatic (**Fig. 9**).

Case 3

A 42-year-old woman presented with 6 months' history of right great toe joint pain. The patient described an axial compression type injury to the joint when shoveling snow.

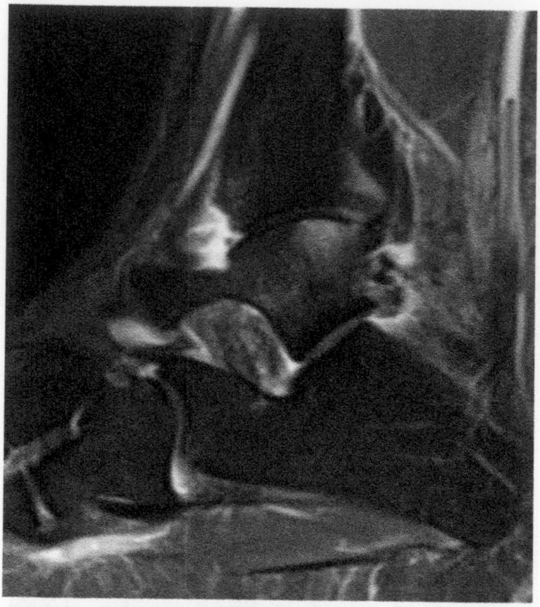

Fig. 4. Lateral MRI T2 image of subchondral contusion.

Clinical examination was positive for joint pain with an axial compression test as well. There was no crepitus or decreased motion appreciated with passive and active flexion and extension of the great toe. Preoperative radiographs (**Fig. 10**) demonstrated a well-defined circumscribed sclerotic defect. MRI demonstrated a hyperintense signal changes within the defect along with hypointense sclerotic ring on the T2-weighted image (**Fig. 11**).

This patient underwent arthrotomy of first metatarsophalangeal joint with cheilectomy and resurfacing of the osteochondral lesion. The lesion was débrided, microfracture performed (**Fig. 12**) and the surface was grafted with an acellular micronized cartilage extracellular matrix secured with fibrin glue (**Fig. 13**). Two years post-procedure, patient is found recovered with episodic residual discomfort but without restriction of activities. No subsequent intervention has been required.

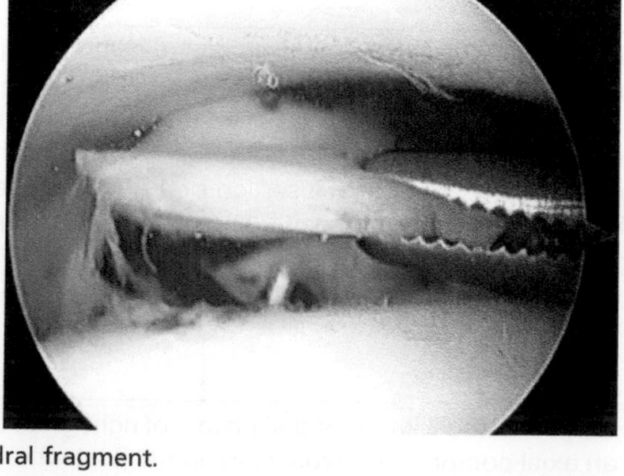

Fig. 5. Osteochondral fragment.

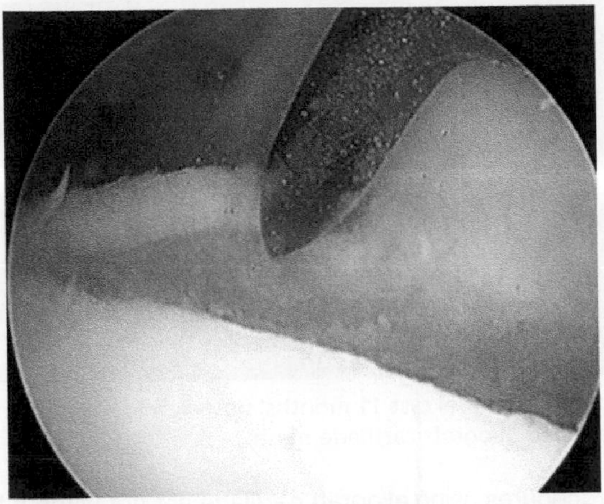

Fig. 6. Débridement followed by microfracture of lesion.

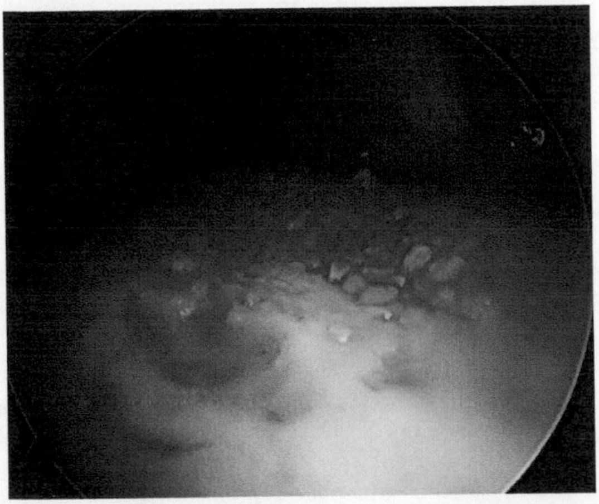

Fig. 7. Final construct with defect filled with micronized cartilage matrix and secured with fibrin glue.

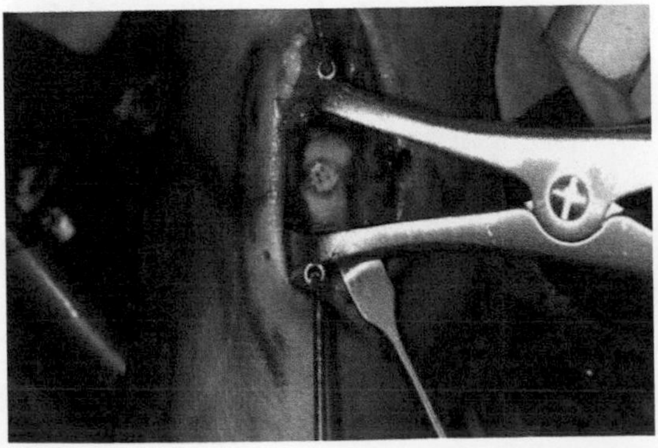

Fig. 8. Application of cryopreserved mesh cartilage secured with central absorbable suture.

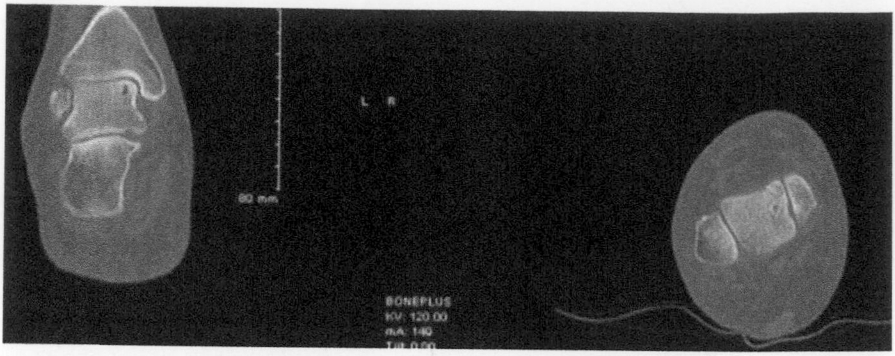

Fig. 9. Asymptomatic subchondral cyst 11 months' post-débridement, bone graft and resurfacing with cryopreserved allograft cartilage mesh.

The identified procedures using allograft cartilage are not without their appreciated real and theoretic shortcomings. To date, there is no ideal method to secure the allograft to enhance integration with the surrounding native cartilage. Techniques to include periosteal flaps, fibrin glue, suturing, and anchors have all been performed but do not ideally create a uniform seamless bond with uninjured native cartilage. Furthermore, these grafts are new and there are no long-term outcomes demonstrating sustainability of the repair to warrant their cost compared with sole

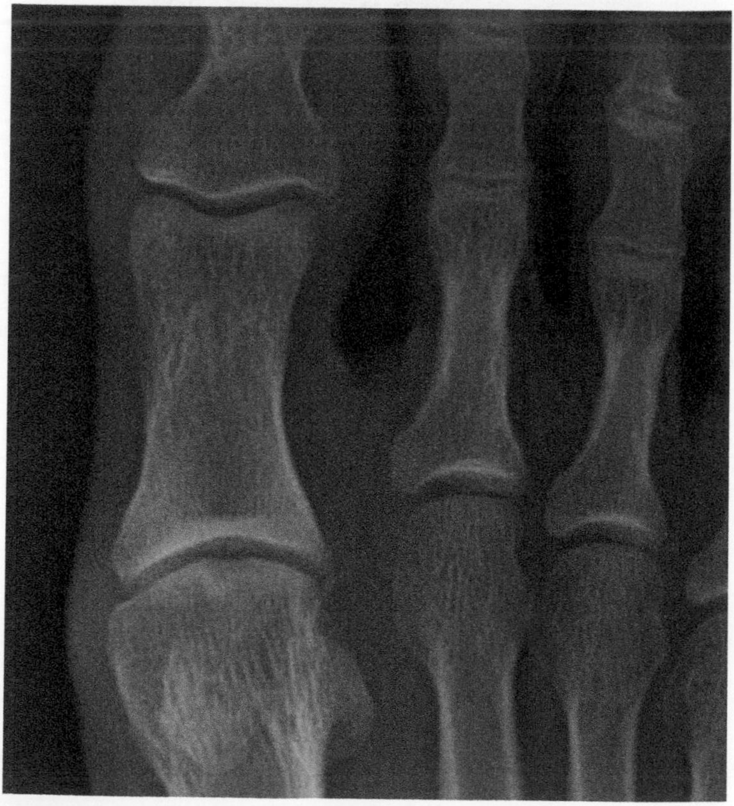

Fig. 10. Central defect of first metatarsal head.

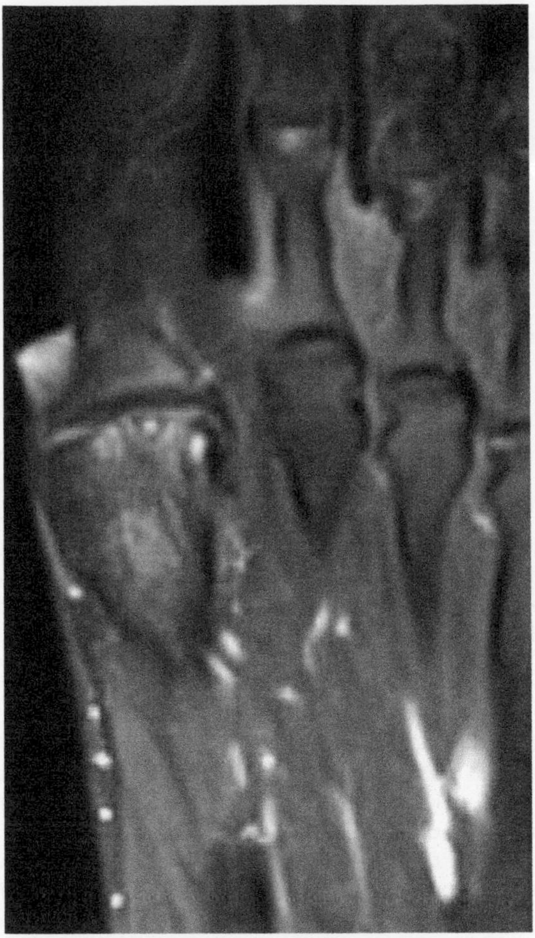

Fig. 11. Hyperintense central defect in subchondral bone of first metatarsal head.

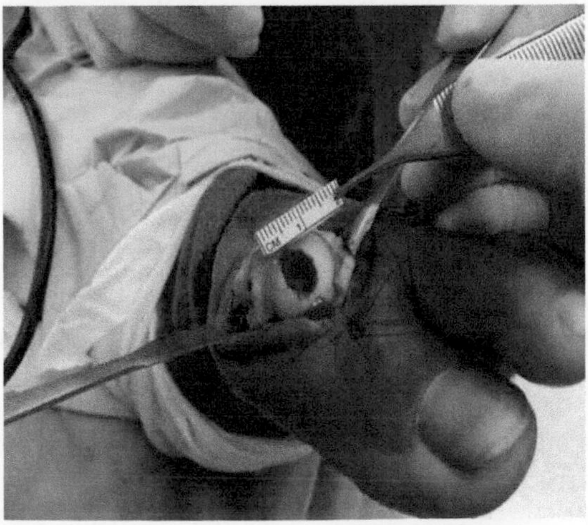

Fig. 12. Débridement and microfracture of osteochondral lesion.

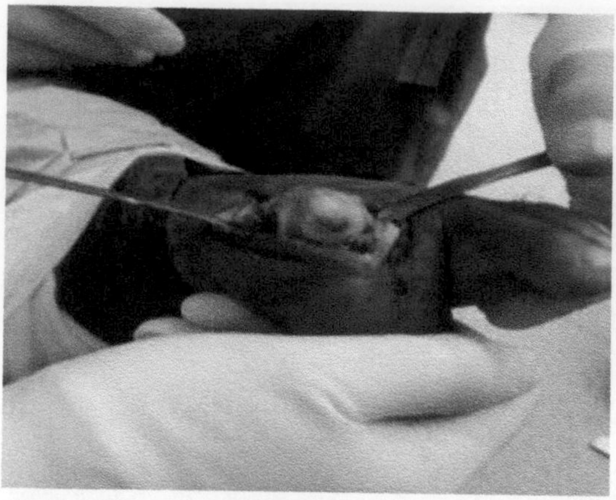

Fig. 13. Resurfaced lesion with micronized cartilage matrix and secured with fibrin glue.

débridement and microfracture. In the short term, it has been the authors' experience that similar outcomes are achieved using allograft cartilage to microfracture but their real benefit of preventing further degeneration or more importantly enhancing restoration of hyaline cartilage remains uncertain.

SUMMARY

Complete repair of articular cartilage damage, whether it is in a toe or an ankle caused by overuse or trauma, is challenging to obtain prearthritic levels of function and pain. Advancements using a variety of allograft tissues and improved surgical techniques have created many new options beyond simply fenestration of a defect with a Kirschner wire. Continued research with improved surgical techniques very close in providing the necessary components for articular repair by using active chondrocytes and a structural and functional extracellular matrix. There remains much to learn, however, to achieve complete cartilage restoration. Further research and advancements in surgical techniques with allograft tissues, for restoration of the native tissue, are necessary to continue to provide better outcomes and improve patient care.

REFERENCES

1. Huber M, Trattnig S, Lintner F. Anatomy, biochemistry, and physiology of articular cartilage. Invest Radiol 2000;35(10):573–80.
2. Landells JW. The reactions of injured human articular cartilage. J Bone Joint Surg Br 1957;39(3):548–62.
3. Pruksakorn D, Pothachareoun P, Klunklin K, et al. Articular cartilage injury treatment: history and basic science review. Orthop Muscul Syst 2012;1:114.
4. Insall J. The Pridie debridement operation for osteoarthritis of the knee. Clin Orthop Relat Res 1974;101:61–7.
5. Steadman JR, Rodkey WG, Singleton SB, et al. Microfracture technique forfull-thickness chondral defects: technique and clinical results. Oper Tech Orthop 1997;7(4):300–4.
6. Farr J, Cole B, Dhawan A, et al. Clinical cartilage restoration: evolution and overview. Clin Orthop Relat Res 2011;469(10):2696–705.

7. Yamashita F, Sakakida K, Suzu F, et al. The transplantation of an autogeneic osteochondral fragment for osteochondritis dissecans of the knee. Clin Orthop Relat Res 1985;201:43–50.
8. Lam CX, Hutmacher DW, Schantz J-T, et al. Evaluation of polycaprolactone scaffold degradation for 6 months in vitro and in vivo. J Biomed Mater Res A 2009; 90(3):906–19.
9. Mintz BR, Cooper JA Jr. Hybrid hyaluronic acid hydrogel/poly(epsilon-caprolactone) scaffold provides mechanically favorable platform for cartilage tissue engineering studies. J Biomed Mater Res A 2014;102(9):2918–26.
10. Oliveira JT, Crawford A, Mundy JM, et al. A cartilage tissue engineering approach combining starch-polycaprolactone fibre mesh scaffolds with bovine articular chondrocytes. J Mater Sci Mater Med 2007;18(2):295–302.
11. Shimozono Y, Yasui Y, Ross AW, et al. Scaffolds based therapy for osteochondral lesions of the talus: a systematic review. World J Orthop 2017;8(10):798–808.
12. Christensen BB, Foldager CB, Jensen J, et al. Poor osteochondral repair by a biomimetic collaged scaffold: 1-to-3-year clincal and radiological follow up. Knee Surg Sports Traumatol Arthrosc 2016;24(7):2380–7.
13. Desai S. Treatment of osteochondral lesions of the talus with marrow stimulation and micronized allograft cartilage matrix: an all-arthroscopic technique. Tech Foot Ankle Surg 2014;13(3):167–73.
14. Liu H, Zhao Z, Clarke RB, et al. Enhanced tissue regeneration potential of juvenile articular cartilage. Am J Sports Med 2013;41(11):2658–67.
15. Vira S, Ramme AJ, Chapman C, et al. Juvenile particulate osteochondral allograft for treatment of osteochondral lesions of the talus: detection of altered repair tissue biochemical composition using 7 Tesla MRI and T2 mapping. J Foot Ankle Surg 2017;56:26–9.
16. Saltzman BM, Lin J, Lee S. Particulated juvenile articular cartilage allograft transplantation for osteochondral talar lesions. Cartilage 2017;8(1):61–72.
17. Van Dyke B, Berlet GC, Daigre JL, et al. First metatarsal head osteochondral defect treatment with particulated juvenile cartilage allograft transplantation: a case series. Foot Ankle Int 2018;39(2):236–41.
18. Csonge L, Bravo D, Newman-Gage H, et al. Banking of osteochondral allografts, part ii. Preservation of chondrocyte viability during long-term storage. Cell Tissue Bank 2002;3(3):161–8.
19. El-Rahidy H, Villacis D, Omar I, et al. Fresh osteochondral allograft for the treatment of cartilage defects of the talus: a retrospective review. J Bone Joint Surg Am 2011;93:1634–40.
20. Hahn DB, Aanstoos ME, Wilkins RM. Osteochondral lesions of the talus treated with fresh talar allografts. Foot Ankle Int 2010;31(4):277–82.
21. Orr JD, Dunn JC, Heida KA, et al. Results and functional outcomes of structural fresh osteochondral allograft transfer for treatment of osteochondral lesions of the talus in a highly active population. Foot Ankle Spec 2017;10(2):125–32.
22. Tan EW, Guyton GP, Miller SD. Cartilage mesh augmentation technique for treatment of osteochondral lesions of the talus. Tech Foot Ankle Surg 2015;14(4): 188–93.

Living Cryopreserved Bone Allograft as an Adjunct for Hindfoot Arthrodesis

Mark K. Magnus, DPM[a], Kelli L. Iceman, DPM[a],
Thomas S. Roukis, DPM, PhD[b,*]

KEYWORDS

- Bone graft • Cellular bone allograft • Mesenchymal stem cell • Nonunion
- Revision surgery

KEY POINTS

- Nonunions are a prevalent and disabling complication of foot and ankle arthrodesis procedures.
- Cellular bone allografts incorporate all 3 essential elements of bone healing while eliminating the commonly associated drawbacks of autografts and traditional allografts.
- Current cellular bone allograft products differ in their source of osteogenic cells, type of scaffolding, and graft composition.
- The available literature demonstrates that cellular bone allografts seem to be safe and effective in hindfoot and ankle arthrodesis procedures.

INTRODUCTION

Hindfoot arthrodesis procedures are commonly performed within a foot and ankle surgeon's practice. Unfortunately, the development of a nonunion remains a prevalent and disabling complication of these surgeries. To improve fusion rates, bone grafts and various biologic supplements are commonly used. This article focuses on the use of bone grafts in hindfoot arthrodesis procedures and the development of orthobiologics, specifically, cellular bone allografts (CBAs). Furthermore, this review aims to provide important considerations with the use of bone grafts as well as practical applications.

Disclosure Statement: T.S. Roukis is a consultant for DePuy Synthes, FH ORTHO, Integra, and Novastep. He owns intellectual property rights with Crossroads Extremity, Novastep, and Stryker. He serves on the *Clinics in Podiatric Medicine & Surgery, Research of Foot & Ankle, Jacobs Foot & Ankle*, and *Diabetic Foot & Ankle* editorial boards, and has received grant/research funding from Gundersen Health System: Medical Foundation.

[a] Gundersen Medical Foundation, Mail Stop: CO3-006A, 1900 South Avenue, La Crosse, WI 54601, USA; [b] Orthopaedic Center, Gundersen Healthcare System, Mail Stop: CO2-006, 1900 South Avenue, La Crosse, WI 54601, USA
* Corresponding author.
E-mail address: tsroukis@gundersenhealth.org

Clin Podiatr Med Surg 35 (2018) 295–310
https://doi.org/10.1016/j.cpm.2018.02.002
podiatric.theclinics.com
0891-8422/18/

HINDFOOT ARTHRODESIS

Arthrodesis is an invaluable procedure for correcting a wide variety of hindfoot pathologies, allowing the surgeon to create a stable, plantigrade foot. National trends in recent years reveal a dramatic increase in the number of foot and ankle arthrodesis procedures performed.[1] This phenomenon is likely secondary to the aging population and associated comorbidities.[1] Considered the gold standard for end-stage arthritis, hindfoot arthrodesis may correct deformities secondary to the following[2]:

- Osteoarthritis,
- Rheumatoid arthritis,
- Traumatic arthritis,
- Charcot arthropathy,
- Long-term instability, and
- Malalignment.

Although the goals of arthrodesis are to reduce pain, enhance function, and provide a better quality of life for the patient, there are several factors that may impede a successful outcome. Such risk factors are either attributed to the patient or the provider[3] (**Table 1**). The patient-specific risk factors compromise vascularity and thereby diminish the delivery of reparative cells and nutrients to the operative site.[4] Previous studies indicate a nonunion rate as high as 40% when performed on these high-risk patients with these aforementioned comorbidities.[5,6]

Patients with symptomatic nonunions often face severe pain and debilitation. In addition, patients may also experience residual psychological and socioeconomic effects, which could lead to potential narcotic dependence or depression.[7] Owing to these complications, foot and ankle surgeons are constantly striving to improve the success rate of arthrodesis procedures with the use of bone grafts and biological augmentation (**Fig. 1**).

BONE GRAFT

Historically, bone grafts were used to fill osseous defects and correct malalignment. More recently, the use of adjunctive bone graft and bone graft substitutes has played a paramount role in hindfoot arthrodesis procedures. Bone grafting aims to increase

Table 1
Risk factors for arthrodesis nonunion

Patient specific	Alcohol abuse Avascular necrosis Diabetes Infection Noncompliance Nonsteroidal antiinflammatories Obesity Old age Osteoporosis Tobacco abuse
Provider specific	Inadequate fixation Insufficient joint preparation Joint surface gapping Poor postoperative protocol

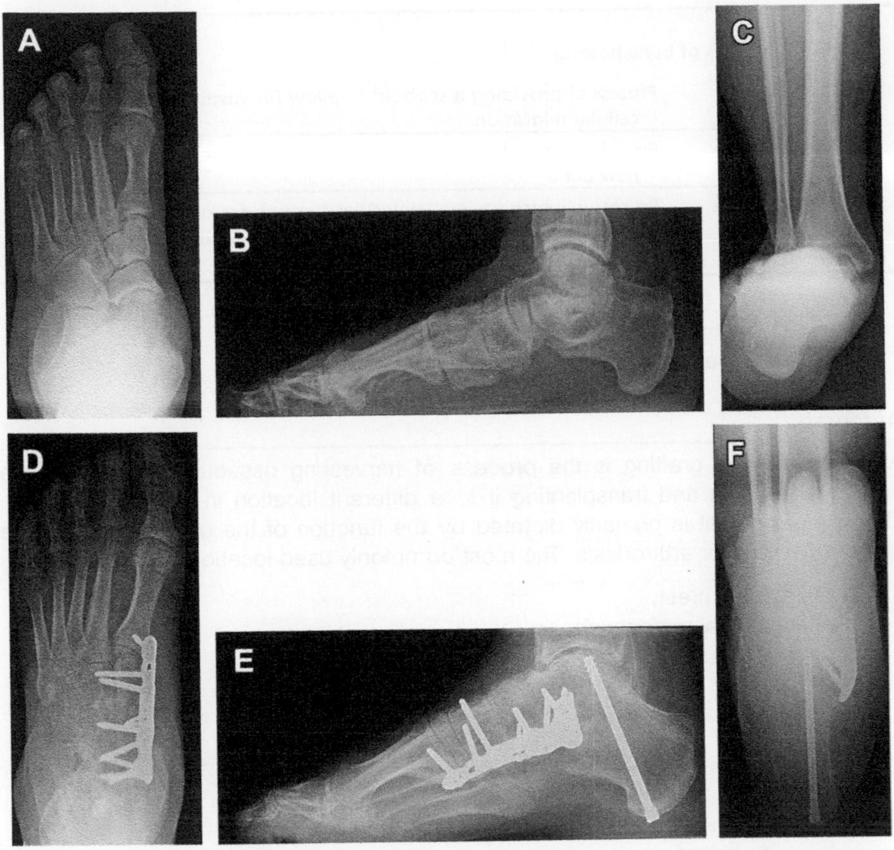

Fig. 1. Preoperative weightbearing anteroposterior (*A*), lateral (*B*), and hindfoot alignment (*C*) views of a patient with multiple comorbidities and stage 3 posterior tibial tendon dysfunction that underwent a medial column and subtalar joint arthrodesis with use of cellular bone matrix with cryopreserved viable bone cells. Final postoperative radiographs (*D–F*) at 1-year follow-up demonstrating mature osseous union and a well-aligned foot.

union rates by stimulating local biology through the 3 essential elements of bone formation: osteoconductive scaffolding, osteoinductive cytokines, and osteogenic cells (**Table 2**).[4]

In regard to bone graft and graft substitutes, an overwhelming amount of options exist (**Fig. 2**). Bone grafts may be grouped by a variety of characteristics, including source (**Table 3**), structure (cancellous, cortical, corticocancellous), biological properties, composition (natural, synthetic), and method of preservation. Unfortunately, there is no consensus regarding a single classification that encompasses all bone grafts. In fact, many grafts are a combination of various properties, sources, or bioactive molecules. To select the appropriate graft, the surgeon must thoroughly consider the following:

- Graft purpose (structural stability, height restoration, fill osseous voids),
- Graft host/recipient location,
- Local perfusion,
- Financial cost,

Table 2
Essential elements of bone healing

Osteoconduction	Process of providing a scaffold to allow for vascular infiltration and cellular migration
Osteogenesis	Provides mesenchymal stem cells and osteoprogenitor cells that form new bone
Osteoinduction	Process in which various molecules (growth factors, matrix proteins, cytokines) induce mesenchymal stem cell and osteoprogenitor cell differentiation into osteoblasts

- Graft advantages and disadvantages, and
- The individual patient.

Autograft

Autologous bone grafting is the process of harvesting osseous tissue from one anatomic location and transplanting it to a different location in the same patient. The site of harvest is primarily dictated by the function of the graft as well as the amount needed for arthrodesis. The most commonly used locations include the:

- Anterior iliac crest,
- Proximal tibial metaphysis,

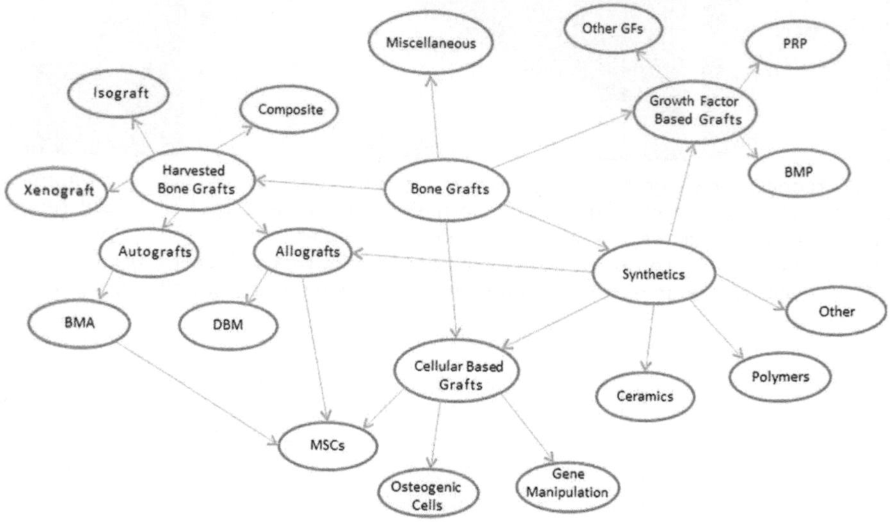

Fig. 2. Bone grafts may be classified as harvested bone grafts, cellular base grafts, synthetics, growth factor–based grafts, and other miscellaneous grafts. Harvested grafts typically include allografts, autografts, xenografts, isografts, and composite grafts. Bone marrow aspirate (BMA) is considered an autograft which also contains MSCs. Depending on the type of allograft, demineralized bone matrix (DBM) and mesenchymal stem cells (MSCs) may be incorporated. Cellular-based grafts are bone grafts that include MSCs, osteogenic cells, and gene manipulated cells. Synthetic grafts may be polymers, ceramics, and various other types. Some bone grafts incorporate allografts on a synthetic scaffold along with other cellular components. Platelet-rich plasma (PRP) and bone morphogenic protein (BMP) are 2 of the most commonly used growth factor (GF)–based grafts, although many other GFs may be used.

Table 3
Sources of bone graft

Autograft	Bone graft transplanted from one site to another in the same patient
Allograft	Bone transplanted from one individual to another genetically unrelated individual of the same species
Composite	Bone grafts made partly from allograft or heterograft and partly autograft
Isograft	Bone graft transplanted form one person to another genetically related individual of the same species
Synthetics	A manufactured graft derived from synthetic materials
Xenograft/heterograft	Bone taken from one species and transplanted into another species

- Distal tibial metaphysis,
- Calcaneus, and the
- Intramedullary cavity of long bones.

Historically, the autograft has been considered the gold standard for stimulating bone repair because it contains the 3 essential elements of bone healing[8] (see **Table 2**). Additionally, autograft is 100% histocompatible, nonimmunogenic, and does not carry the risk of disease transmission.[9,10]

Cancellous grafts are commonly used in foot and ankle surgery. These grafts contain osteogenic cells, as well as a lattice of trabecular bone that is highly angiogenic and readily incorporates into the host bone.[10] However, these grafts lack structural integrity and are not ideal to sustain compressive loads when used in isolation.[10] Cortical grafts provide excellent structural stability; however, they are slow to incorporate into host bone because the cortex contains minimal osteogenic properties.[10] Corticocancellous grafts combine both the osteogenic and osteoconductive properties from cancellous grafts with the added stability of cortical grafts.[10] These grafts are typically obtained from the anterior iliac crest and may provide up to 3 cortices.

Although autografts may have once been considered the gold standard, they are not without their own set of limitations. The incidence of complications and postoperative morbidity after harvesting an autograft has been reported as high as 23%.[11] Major complications are those that cause extensive injury or require additional medical treatment. Complications that do not cause long-term disability or significantly alter the patient's treatment course are considered minor complications (**Table 4**).[4,8,10,12]

When selecting a bone graft for an arthrodesis procedure, it is also imperative to consider the graft quality. Studies have shown that autograft donor sites are not equal with respect to osteogenic properties.[13,14] Chiodo and colleagues[13] performed a histologic study that compared bone graft samples from the iliac crest and the proximal tibia. Their results revealed significantly more active hematopoietic marrow in the iliac crest samples, whereas proximal tibial grafts contained more quiescent fat.[13] Hyer and colleagues[14] demonstrated marrow aspirates from the iliac crest contained a higher concentration of mesenchymal stem osteoprogenitor cells compared with the distal tibia and calcaneus. These findings suggest that alternative autograft sites (ie, tibia, calcaneus) may have limited cellular healing potential and, therefore, may not be the most effective autograft sources. Furthermore, the quality of the autograft is also influenced by the patient's age, metabolic abnormalities, and tobacco use.[9] With the need for a reliable and reproducible bone graft without the associated

Table 4 Complications associated with autograft	
Major complications	Deep donor site infection/hematoma Donor site fracture Gait disturbance Incisional hernia Major neurovascular injury
Minor complications	Donor site pain Sensory nerve injury Superficial hematoma/seroma Superficial infection Wounding
Other considerations	Extended anesthetic time Increased blood loss Limited quantities

complications and postoperative morbidity of an autograft, alternative graft sources and materials have become increasingly popular among foot and ankle surgeons.

Allograft

Allogeneic bone grafting refers to the process of harvesting osseous tissue from one individual and transplanting it into a different individual of the same species. Clear advantages to this form of bone grafting are the lack of donor site morbidity and reduced surgical time. Unlike autografts, allografts have a relative unlimited supply and come in a variety of different shapes, sizes, types, and forms (**Table 5**). Depending on the type used, some allografts may retain all 3 essential elements of bone healing, whereas others may only contribute osteoconductive properties.

- Fresh allografts commonly contain osteogenic viable cells, osteoinductive cytokines, and an osteoconductive scaffold.[15] These grafts retain their biological properties because there is limited procurement and processing.[15]
- Fresh frozen allografts typically retain their structural stability as well as contain osteoconductive and osteoinductive properties.[16] However, the degree of osteoinductive potential depends on the cryopreservation techniques (conventional freezing, deep freezing, or liquid nitrogen freezing) and storage methods.[15]
- Freeze-dried allografts are used for their osteoconductive properties. These grafts are initially frozen and then undergo cryodesiccation (a dehydration

Table 5
Allograft bone types and forms

Types	Forms
Fresh allograft Fresh frozen allograft Freeze-dried allograft Demineralized bone matrix	Chips (cancellous, corticocancellous) Cortical bone segments Custom shapes Granules Injectables Paste Putty Sheets Strips

process under vacuum pressure).[15] This processing alters the structural integrity of the bone while also stripping the graft of viable cells and infectious agents.[15]

- Demineralized bone matrix (DBM)/allograft provides enhanced osteoinductive properties. Hydrochloric acid demineralizes the bone matrix and removes inorganic minerals.[15] The remaining graft constituents are the collagen matrix and bioactive products (bone morphogenic protein and various growth factors).[17] DBM does provide osteoconductive properties; however, it lacks structural support and, therefore, is often used in conjunction with other grafts.

There are a fair amount of clinical studies that compare the safety and efficacy between the use of allografts and autografts within the foot and ankle literature. Müller and colleagues[18] performed a systematic review that compared autograft and allograft union rates in 928 hindfoot arthrodesis and osteotomy procedures. The authors concluded that allografts and autografts have equivalent incorporation rates.[18] Tricot and colleagues[19] compared the use of combination grafts (autograft with DBM vs allograft with DBM and BMA) in 115 hindfoot and ankle arthrodesis procedures. The study revealed there was no significant difference between the 2 groups in terms of union rate, time to fusion, or revision rate.[19] Overall, the literature is promising and suggests that allogenic bone grafts are a viable option for surgical reconstructive procedures.

Although there are many benefits of using allografts, there are also disadvantages. As mentioned, depending on the type of allograft and the sterilization techniques used, allografts rarely incorporate all 3 essential elements of bone healing.[8] Not only does the often-used irradiation sterilization process diminish the graft's biological properties, but it has also been shown to reduce the structural integrity of the graft as well.[8] Although allografts may have an "off-the-shelf" convenience, they are also more costly than autografts—an important consideration given the increasing costs of health care. Last, allografts carry the risk of infectious disease transmission.[8,12] This risk, however, has substantially decreased as a result of strict regulations enforced by the US Food and Drug Administration and the American Associated Tissue Banks, as well as the graft sterilization processes.[15] The estimated risk of human immunodeficiency virus transmission is 1 in 2.8 billion with use of DBM and freeze-dried allografts.[20] Although the incidence of hepatitis C and other viral disease transmission is unknown, it is also believed to be exceedingly rare.[21]

Ongoing research continues to advance technology in the hopes of overcoming the limitations of autologous and allogenic bone grafts. To this regard, the development of orthobiologics aims to use cell-based therapies and biomaterials as an adjunct or an alternative to traditional grafting methods.

CELLULAR BONE ALLOGRAFT

As the name implies, CBAs are composed of a structural allogenic bone matrix with a viable cellular component. These grafts aim to incorporate all 3 essential elements of bone healing while eliminating the commonly associated drawbacks of autografts and traditional allografts. Although numerous CBA products are available, virtually all these products incorporate mesenchymal stem cells (MSCs).

Mesenchymal Stem Cells

There is considerable potential with the use of stem cell research to aid in regenerative and reparative therapies. Stem cells are undifferentiated cells that possess the capability of self-replication. Sources of stem cells are either adult somatic stem cells or embryonic stem cells. Many ethical and political issues occur with the use of embryonic stem cells and, therefore, research has focused on somatic stem cells and their potential clinical applications. Somatic stem cells are found in many organs and tissues throughout the body. MSCs are a type of somatic stem cell that are commonly isolated from the bone marrow; however, they may also be harvested from other sources such as the teeth, skin, umbilical cord, and adipose tissue.[22]

MSCs are considered multipotent; they retain the ability to self-replicate and also differentiate into the cells of the mesoderm (bone, cartilage, fat, muscle, nerve).[22] Their fate to become any specific cell is determined by both intrinsic and local environmental factors (spatial organization, mechanical forces, cytokines, and nutrients).[22] Under specific conditions an osteoprogenitor cell, an MSC destined to undergo osteogenesis, will differentiate into osteoblasts and form bone.

It was long believed that MSCs were nonimmunogenic, allowing them to be transplanted across major histocompatibility barriers without concern for host rejection.[23] MSCs were assumed to avoid immune system recognition and T-cell activation owing to their lack the major histocompatibility complex II and accessory molecules (CD40, CD40L, CD80, and CD86).[9] However, recent studies have demonstrated donor MSCs elicit a humoral and cellular host immune response.[22,23] Therefore, it is argued that MSCs are not truly nonimmunogenic but should instead be considered "immune evasive."[23] More specifically, MSCs possess innate paracrine and autocrine capabilities, which enable them to secrete immunomodulatory factors to influence their local environment.[22] These signals have been shown to suppress the host immune response, thereby allowing donor MSCs to temporarily prevent rejection.[23] Some studies contend that there is such a limited persistence of donor MSCs after implantation that the time for differentiation and actual incorporation into the host tissues would be unlikely.[23,24] Therefore, conventional wisdom suggests the true therapeutic effect of donor MSCs relies on these secreted immunomodulatory factors and their ability to recruit host MSCs and other supportive cells, rather than their innate pluripotent potential.

Cellular Bone Allograft Processing and Preservation

The majority of CBAs use cadaveric bone for harvesting MSCs. Initially, cadaveric bone samples undergo rigorous screening through the US Food and Drug Administration and American Associated Tissue Banks and then are harvested from the donor within a narrow window of time.[9] The MSCs are readily available and well-adhered to the trabeculae of cancellous bone.[9] Other nutrients and cellular components imperative for bone healing are also located within the harvested bone.[9] Depending on the type of bone graft, the cortical and cancellous bone components are processed individually and then recombined to create the final product.[9] During the processing, donor immunogens are removed and the native MSCs remain. Once the graft has been generated, it is combined with a cryoprotectant solution and frozen. Cryopreservation is used to freeze bone in a controlled manner so that water crystals do not damage viable cells or cause them to undergo apoptosis.[25] This method has been shown to recover more than 95% of cells while retaining their biologic capacity after the thawing process.[26]

Once a specific CBA product is selected, it must be prepared before implantation. Although each product has its own specific preparation process, a majority of available products follow a similar method. Most products must first undergo a thawing process for a designated period of time in a sterile basin containing saline that is usually warmed to physiologic temperatures (37°C ± 2°C). Once completely thawed, the cryopreservation solution is decanted. Next, the graft is rinsed with an irrigant solution (sterile saline, lactated Ringers, etc), which is also decanted before implantation. It should be noted that the cell viability after the thawing process can vary between products and thus must be coordinated appropriately with the surgical procedure being performed.

Clinical Applications

Reported nonunion rates for hindfoot and ankle arthrodesis are roughly 10% to 15%.[27] As discussed, the nonunion rates may be substantially higher depending on patient comorbidities and risk factors. Recent literature has shown promise with use of CBAs as an adjunctive bone graft. Multiple studies have shown equal, if not superior, union rates in foot and ankle arthrodesis procedures.

- Hollawell[28] described a case series where 20 patients underwent a subtalar joint or an ankle fusion using CBAs (Osteocel Plus, NuVasive, Inc, San Diego, CA). The reported union rate was 100% with a mean time to fusion of 13.5 weeks.[28] The author concluded that the product was a safe and effective method for bone healing in foot and ankle arthrodesis procedures.[28]
- Jones and colleagues[2] performed a prospective study using CBAs (Trinity Evolution, Orthofix, Inc, Lewisville, TX) in hindfoot and/or ankle fusions. At the end of the 1-year study, 86.6% of the 129 arthrodesis procedures had successfully fused.[2] The authors found no differences in union rates between the higher risk subjects and normal patients.[2] They concluded that CBAs were safe and effective to achieve fusion in patients with compromised bone healing and that CBAs may be a valuable alternative to autografts.[2]
- Scott and Hyer[29] reported a 90% union rate in 20 high-risk diabetic patients who underwent hindfoot or ankle fusions with the use of CBAs (Osteocel Plus, NuVasive, Inc).[29] The mean time to fusion was 11.6 weeks. The authors concluded that CBAs played a vital role in successful hindfoot and ankle fusions within high-risk patients.[29]
- Rush[30] retrospectively reviewed 23 patients who underwent revision foot and/or ankle surgery with the use of CBAs (Trinity Multipotential Cellular Bone Matrix, Orthofix, Inc). The mean time to fusion was 10.4 weeks with a 91.3% union rate.[30] There were no reported complications associated with the use of CBAs and no graft rejection was identified.[30] The authors concluded that CBAs provided a safe, viable alternative to autografts in the setting of revision surgery with satisfactory clinical and radiographic outcomes.[30]
- Clements[31] reported a case using a CBA (Osteocel Plus, NuVasive, Inc) in 1 patient who developed avascular necrosis of the talus complicated by septic arthritis. This patient underwent a staged procedure that ultimately resulted in a talectomy and tibiocalcaneal arthrodesis.[31] Solid fusion was reported at 12 weeks.[31] The authors concluded that CBAs seem to be a viable alternative for surgical reconstructive cases where there has been substantial bone loss and prior infection.[31]
- Dekker and colleagues[4] reported an 83% union rate in 23 high-risk patients who underwent foot or ankle fusions with the use of CBAs (Map3, RTI Surgical Inc, Alachua, FL). The findings suggested the presence of diabetes was the only independent risk factor for nonunion development.[4] The authors concluded this product was a successful and potential alternative graft substitute for arthrodesis procedures in high-risk patients.[4]
- Anderson and colleagues[32] compared the use of CBAs (varying products) and proximal tibial autografts in 85 patients. The authors found an 84.1% union rate in the CBA group and a 95.1% in the autograft group.[32] The mean time to fusion was 13.1 weeks and 11.0 weeks for the CBA and the autograft groups,

respectively.[32] The authors concluded there was no statistically significant difference between the 2 groups in terms of union rates; however, the CBA group showed a statistically significant delay in time to fusion.[32]

- Loveland and colleagues[33] performed a comparative retrospective study between CBAs (Trinity Evolution and Trinity ELITE, Orthofix, Inc) in 141 foot and/or ankle arthrodesis procedures. At 12 months of follow-up, the fusion rate was 93.3% and 85.7% for the Trinity Evolution and Trinity ELITE groups,

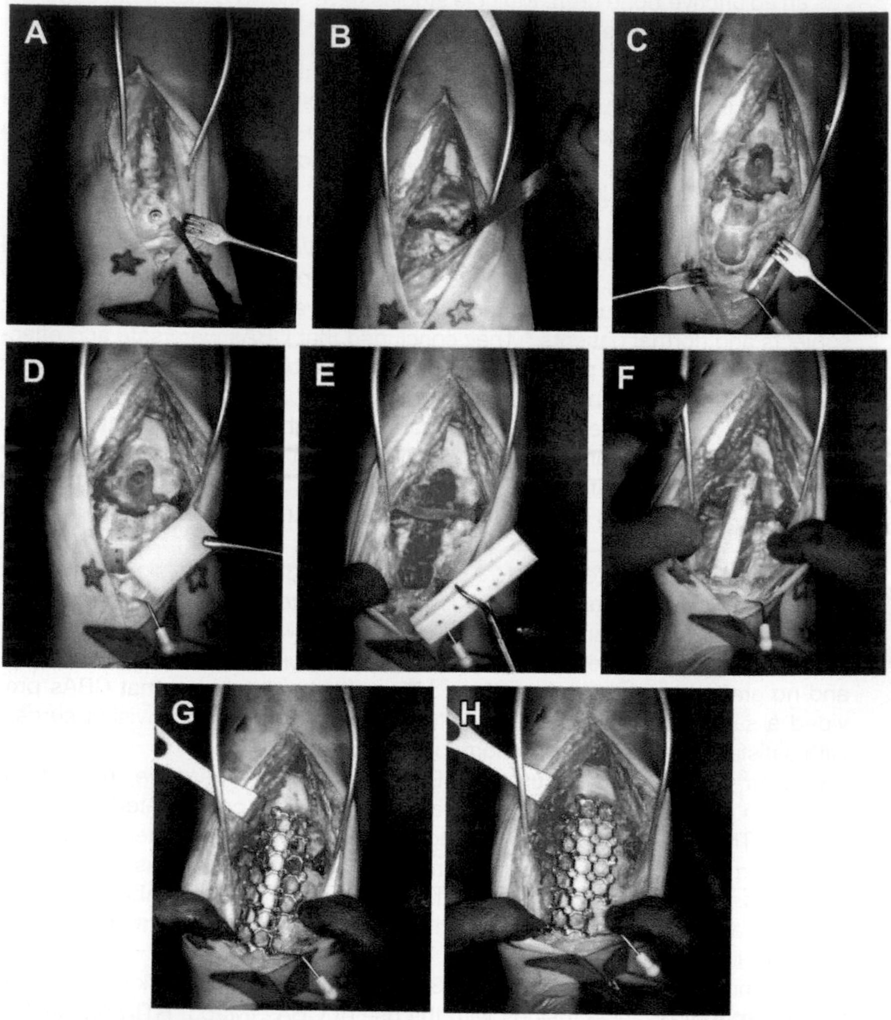

Fig. 3. Failed talonavicular arthrodesis for treatment of a prior navicular fracture and avascular necrosis. Fibrotic scar tissue with deep retained hardware (*A*) and resection of the nonunion (*B*). Owing to extensive bone loss, a trough was created through the talar neck, navicular, medial cuneiform, and first metatarsal (*C*). Demineralized cancellous bone sheet (*D*) and cellular bone matrix with cryopreserved viable bone cells was used to fill the void. The fibula allograft was rehydrated, fenestrated (*E*), and press fit into the trough (*F*). A dorsal bridge plate was used to overlay the construct (*G*). Distal tibial bone marrow aspirate was mixed with cancellous allograft bone chips and impacted into the remaining defects about the medial column (*H*).

respectively.[33] No significant difference was found between the 2 groups in terms of union rate.[33] The patient's clinical risk factors were also not found to cause any significant difference in terms of union rates.[33]

- Coetzee and colleagues[34] performed a prospective, randomized study comparing tibial autologenous bone graft to CBAs (Allostem, AlloSource, Centennial, CO) in subtalar joint arthrodesis procedures in 110 patients. The authors determined the arthrodesis rates were equivocal and there were no statistically significant differences in outcome scores between the 2 groups.[34]

Overall, the literature suggests that CBAs seem to be a safe, effective, and viable option for hindfoot/ankle arthrodesis procedures. However, the lack of standardization in fusion techniques, the type and amount of CBA used, clinical protocols, and patient populations makes comparing results across studies difficult. Furthermore, the lack of randomization, absence of control groups, and small sample sizes makes it challenging to determine the efficacy of the CBA products. Non–industry-sponsored, higher level studies with larger patient populations, long-term follow-up, and cost–benefit analyses are needed.

Another clinical application of CBAs includes using them in combination with other grafting techniques. **Fig. 3** shows a failed talonavicular arthrodesis for the treatment of a prior navicular fracture and avascular necrosis. The revision surgery required removal of the deep retained hardware (see **Fig. 3**A) and resection of the nonunion (see **Fig. 3**B). Owing to extensive bone loss, a trough in the talar neck, navicular, medial cuneiform, and first metatarsal was made to allow placement of a structural, freeze-dried fibular allograft (see **Fig. 3**C). To fill the void at the talonavicular joint, another allograft (CONFORM Flex, DePuy Synthes, Raynham, MA) and CBA product (ViviGen Formable, DePuy Synthes) was used (see **Fig. 3**D). The fibula allograft was then rehydrated, fenestrated, and press fit into the trough (see **Fig. 3**E, F). A dorsal

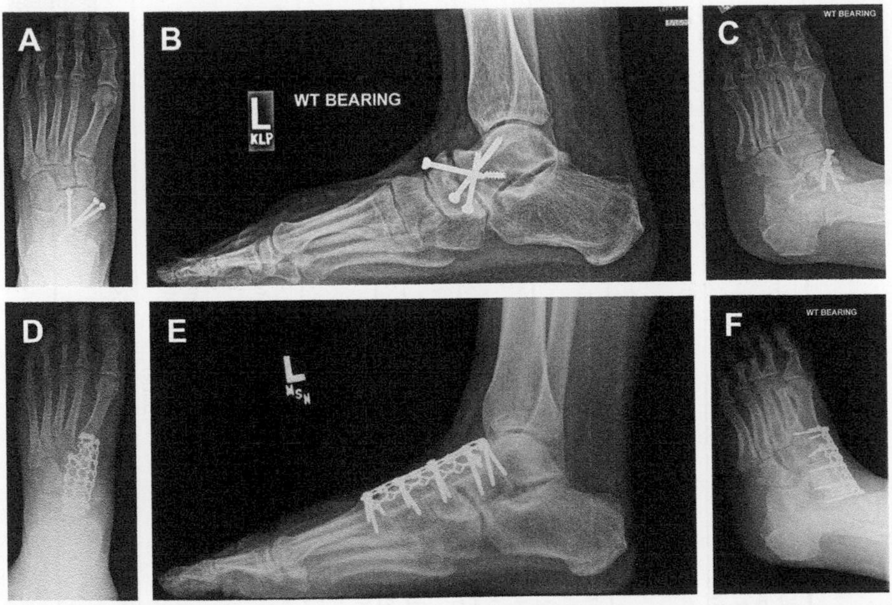

Fig. 4. Preoperative anteroposterior (*A*), lateral (*B*), and oblique (*C*) views of a talonavicular joint nonunion that underwent a medial column fusion (shown in **Fig. 3**). Final postoperative radiographs (*D–F*) at 6-months follow-up demonstrating mature osseous union.

Table 6
Cellular bone allograft products

Product	Allostem[35]	Arthrocell[36]	Bio4[37]	Cellentra Advanced Allograft[38]	Map3[39]	Osteocel Plus[40]	Ovation[41]	Trinity Evolution (Elite)[42]	V92[43]	Vivigen (Formable)[44]
Manufacturer	Allosource	Arthrex	Stryker	Zimmer Biomet	RTI	Nuvasive	Osiris	Orthofix	Paragon	Depuy Synthes
Average age of donor at harvest (y)	50	15–55				18–44		30	15–55	<60
MSC source	Cadaveric adipose tissue	Cadaveric vertebral body				Cadaveric bone	Live donor placenta chorion layer	Cadaveric bone		Cadaveric iliac crest, femoral head, talus
Total cellular concentration (cells/mL)	66,255	150,000	600,000	250,000		250,000	400,000	250,000	150,000	>16,666
No. of viable osteogenic cells (cells/mL)										>16,000 cells/mL
Storage temperature (°C)	(−)80	(−)65		(−)70		(−)80	(−)75–85	(−)70–80	(−)65–80	(−)70
Shelf life (mo)	60	24		18		60		12	24	6
Time for cell viability once thawed (h)		4	1	4		4		2	2	2
Osteoconductive carrier	DBM	Mineralized and DBM particulate (cortical shavings, crushed cancellous chips, microparticulate bone)	DBM, bone chips, cancellous bone	DBM, cancellous bone matrix	DBM, corticocancellous bone chips	DBM		DBM	DBM, microparticulate, cortical, cancellous bone	DBM, corticocancellous chips
Cell populations	MSCs	MIAMI cells, OPCs, MSCs	MSCs, OPCs, osteoblasts	MSCs, OPC, pre-osteoblasts	MAPC	MSCs, OPCs		MSCs, OPCs	MIAMI cells, MSCs	Bone cells (osteoblasts, osteocytes, bone lining cells)

Abbreviations: DBM, demineralized bone matrix; MAPC, multipotent adult progenitor cells; MIAMI, marrow-isolated adult multilineage inducible cells; MSC, mesenchymal stem cell; OPC, osteoprogenitor cell.

mesh bridge plate (Variable Angle LCP Mesh Plate 2.4/2.7, DePuy Synthes) was then customized to increase the stability of the construct (see **Fig. 3**G). Autograft, in the form of distal tibial BMA, was obtained and then mixed with cancellous allograft bone chips. These were impacted into the osseous defects about the medial column (see **Fig. 3**H). **Fig. 4** displays the preoperative and 5-month postoperative radiographs. This is an excellent example of how CBAs may be used in conjunction with other forms of bone grafts to provide the 3 essential elements of bone healing, as well as structural stability, in complex arthrodesis procedures.

Cellular Bone Allograft Considerations

Despite the shared characteristics of CBAs, the products currently available often differ in their source of MSCs, type of scaffolding, and composition of active cells (**Table 6**).[35–44] Although a majority of commercially available CBAs use harvested MSCs from cadaveric bone, products such as Allostem (AllosSource, Centennial, CO) and Ovation (Osiris Therapeutics, Columbia, MD) use cadaveric adipose tissue and the placental chorion layer from a live donor, respectively.[35,41] Regardless of where the MSCs are harvested, each CBA product uses a proprietary blend of corticocancellous chips and mineralized/demineralized bone to serve as an osteoconductive carrier of the active cells.

The main difference between the products is the unique population of osteogenic cells and cytokines. In particular, 2 products, Arthrocell (Arthrex, Naples, FL) and V92 (Paragon 28, Englewood, CO), advocate the use of marrow-isolated adult multilineage inducible cells, which have expanded differentiation potential (ie, endoderm, mesoderm, and ectoderm), similar to embryonic stem cells.[36,43,45] In contrast, other companies favor the use of narrowed MSC lineages specifically destined for the osteogenic pathway because the formation of bone is directly proportional to the amount of osteoblasts available, which in turn is directly proportional to the number of MSCs committed to the osteogenic lineage pathway. To this point, ViviGen (DePuy Synthes) was developed with only osteogenic cells (osteoblasts, osteocytes, bone lining cells).[44] In contrast with undifferentiated MSCs, bone cells are fully differentiated and are committed to the formation of osseous tissue. Thus, ViviGen (DePuy Synthes) avoids the erroneous production of cartilage and muscle by providing lineage-committed bone cells.[44]

Perhaps the most critical concern when deciding between products is the number of active cells available before and after the preparation process. Although several companies emphasize vast quantities of MSCs and other osteogenic cells, only a select few products actually disclose the number of surviving cells after the thawing and preparation processes (see **Table 6**). Unfortunately, the current literature lacks an accepted standard number of MSCs needed to promote bony healing in the setting of arthrodesis, adding another layer of complexity to the issue. Future studies are needed to provide CBA guidelines regarding product contents, which will allow transparency between the manufactures and surgeons.

SUMMARY

Hindfoot arthrodesis is a common procedure for treating pathology varying from end-stage osteoarthritis to Charcot arthropathy. The main goal of the procedure is to reduce pain, correct deformity, and enhance the patient's function. The success of the surgery, however, can be devastated by the presence of a nonunion. When symptomatic, nonunions can become painfully debilitating, as well as a socioeconomic and psychological burden on the patient. To mitigate the risk of nonunion, surgeons have resorted to using bone graft as an adjunct to arthrodesis procedures.

Not all bone grafts are created equal, with each type contributing a unique set of biological properties. Once considered the gold standard, autografts provide the 3 essential elements of bone healing, but can be associated with unwanted postoperative morbidity. Allografts avoid the potential complications of autograft harvesting while providing structural support in a variety of shapes and sizes. The major disadvantage of the most commonly used allografts is their lack of osteogenic and osteoinductive capabilities.

When considering the ideal bone graft, the following properties are crucial:

- Immunologic and histologic compatibility,
- Osteoconductive scaffolding,
- Osteoinductive cytokines,
- Viable potential osteogenic cells, and
- Avoidance of donor site morbidity/complications.

The desire to find an alternative to autografts has led to the creation of CBAs. More specifically, CBAs possess all the essential elements of bone healing without the donor site morbidity and complications, virtually making them the ideal bone graft. CBAs take advantage of a structural allogenic bone matrix with an added viable cellular component through the use of MSCs. Under certain conditions an MSC can be induced to differentiate into osteoblasts and form bone. This unique feature provides CBAs an advantage in compromised patients with several comorbidities and other risk factors for nonunion. It must be noted that the use of CBAs alone does not guarantee a desirable result, nor will it ever replace the importance of proper joint preparation and surgical technique.

Although this is a fast developing field, there is a need for further research regarding the use and efficacy of these products. Prospective randomized control trials are needed, as well as studies that compare successful fusion rates between CBAs and traditional grafting techniques. However, the available literature shows promise with the use of CBAs to enhance bony healing. For the time being, current studies demonstrate that CBAs seem to be safe and effective in hindfoot and ankle arthrodesis procedures.

REFERENCES

1. Best M, Buller L, Miranda A. National trends in foot and ankle arthrodesis: 17-year analysis of the National Survey of Ambulatory Surgery and National Hospital Discharge Survey. J Foot Ankle Surg 2015;54:1037–41.
2. Jones C, Loveland J, Atkinson B, et al. Prospective, multicenter evaluation of allogenic bone matrix containing viable osteogenic cells in foot and/or ankle arthrodesis. Foot Ankle Int 2015;36:1129–37.
3. Thevendran G, Younger A, Pinney S. Current concepts review: risk factors for nonunions in foot and ankle arthrodesis. Foot Ankle Int 2012;33:1031–40.
4. Dekker T, White P, Adams S. Efficacy of a cellular allogeneic bone graft in foot and ankle arthrodesis procedures. Foot Ankle Int 2016;21:855–61.
5. DiGiovanni C, Lin S, Baumhauer J, et al. Recombinant human platelet-derived growth factor-BB and beta-tricalcium phosphate (rhPDGF-BB/b-TCP): an alternative to autogenous bone graft. J Bone Joint Surg Am 2013;95:1184–92.
6. Chahal J, Stephen D, Bulmer B, et al. Factors associated with outcome after subtalar arthrodesis. J Orthop Trauma 2006;20:555–61.

7. Catanzariti A, Moore K. Complication management: nonunions. In: Lee M, Grossman J, editors. Complications in foot and ankle surgery. 1st edition. Cham (Switzerland): Springer International Publishing; 2017. p. 29–53.
8. Roberts T, Rosenbaum A. Bone grafts, bone substitutes and orthobiologics the bridge between basic science and clinical advancements in fracture healing. Organogenesis 2012;8:114–24.
9. Grabowski G, Robertson R. Bone allograft with mesenchymal stem cells: a critical review of the literature. Hard Tissue 2013;2:20.
10. Miller C, Chiodo C. Autologous bone graft in foot and ankle surgery. Foot Ankle Clin 2016;21:825–37.
11. Ahlmann E, Patzakis M, Roidis N, et al. Comparison of anterior and posterior iliac crest bone grafts in terms of harvest-site morbidity and functional outcomes. J Bone Joint Surg Am 2002;84-A:716–20.
12. Nandi S, Roy S, Mukherjee P, et al. Orthopaedic applications of bone graft & graft substitutes: a review. Indian J Med Res 2010;132:15–30.
13. Chiodo C, Hahne J, Wilson M, et al. Histological differences in iliac and tibial bone graft. Foot Ankle Int 2010;31:418–22.
14. Hyer C, Berlet G, Bussewitz B, et al. Quantitative assessment of the yield of osteoblastic connective tissue progenitors in bone marrow aspirate from the iliac crest, tibia and calcaneus. J Bone Joint Surg Am 2013;95:1312–6.
15. Cook E, Cook J. Bone graft substitutes and allografts for reconstruction of the foot and ankle. Clin Podiatr Med Surg 2009;26:589–605.
16. Wee J, Thevendran G. The role of orthobiologics in foot and ankle surgery: allogenic bone grafts and bone graft substitutes. EFORT Open Rev 2017;2:272–80.
17. Arner J, Santrock R. A historical review of common bone graft materials in foot and ankle surgery. Foot Ankle Spec 2014;7:143–51.
18. Müller M, Frank A, Briel M, et al. Substitutes of structural and non-structural autologous bone grafts in hindfoot arthrodesis and osteotomies: a systematic review. BMC Musculoskelet Disord 2013;14:59.
19. Tricot M, Deleu PA, Detrembleur C, et al. Clinical assessment of 115 cases of hindfoot fusion with two different types of graft: allograft+DBMbone marrow aspirate versus autograft+DBM. Orthop Traumatol Surg Res 2017;103:697–702.
20. Russo R, Scarborough N. Inactivation of viruses in demineralized bone matrix. Presented at the FDA workshop on tissue transplantation and reproductive tissue. Bethesda (MD), June 20–21, 1995.
21. Joyce M. Safety and FDA regulations for musculoskeletal allografts: perspective of an orthopaedic surgeon. Clin Orthop Relat Res 2005;435:22–30.
22. Skovrlj B, Guzman J, Al Maaieh M, et al. Cellular bone matrices: viable stem cell-containing bone graft substitutes. Spine J 2014;14:2763–72.
23. Ankrum J, Ong JF, Karp J. Mesenchymal stem cells: immune evasive, not immune privileged. Nat Biotechnol 2014;32:252–60.
24. von Bahr L, Batsis I, Moll G, et al. Analysis of tissues following mesenchymal stromal cell therapy in humans indicates limited long-term engraftment and no ectopic tissue formation. Stem Cells 2012;30:1575–8.
25. Simonson O, Domogatskaya A, Volchkov P, et al. The safety of human pluripotent stem cells in clinical treatment. Ann Med 2015;47:370–80.
26. Bruder S, Jaiswal N, Haynesworth S. Growth kinetics, self-renewal, and osteogenic potential of purified human mesenchymal stem cells during extensive subcultivation and following cryopreservation. J Cell Biochem 1997;64:278–94.
27. Davies M, Rosenfeld P, Stavrou P, et al. A comprehensive review of subtalar arthrodesis. Foot Ankle Int 2007;28:295–7.

28. Hollawell S. Allograft cellular bone matrix as an alternative to autograft in hindfoot and ankle fusion procedures. J Foot Ankle Surg 2012;51:222–5.
29. Scott R, Hyer C. Role of cellular allograft containing mesenchymal stem cells in high-risk foot and ankle reconstructions. J Foot Ankle Surg 2013;52:32–5.
30. Rush S. Trinity evolution: mesenchymal stem cell allografting in foot and ankle surgery. Foot Ankle Spec 2010;3:140–3.
31. Clements J. Use of allograft cellular bone matrix in multistage talectomy with tibiocalcaneal arthrodesis: a case report. J Foot Ankle Surg 2012;51:83–6.
32. Anderson J, Boone J, Hansen M, et al. Ankle arthrodesis fusion rates for mesenchymal stem cell bone allograft versus proximal tibia autograft. J Foot Ankle Surg 2014;53:683–6.
33. Loveland J, Waldorff E, He D, et al. A retrospective clinical comparison of two allogeneic bone matrices containing viable osteogenic cells in patients undergoing foot and/or ankle arthrodesis. J Stem Cell Res Ther 2017;7:405.
34. Coetzee J, Myerson M, Anderson J. The use of allostem in subtalar fusions. Foot Ankle Clin 2016;21:863–8.
35. AlloStem Cellular Bone Allograft. In: AlloSource. 2016. Available at: http://www.allosource.org/products/allostem-cellular-bone-allograft/. Accessed November 25, 2017.
36. ArthroCell Bone Allograft. In: Arthrex. Arthrex Arthrocell. 2017. Available at: https://www.arthrex.com/orthobiologics/arthrocell. Accessed November 25, 2017.
37. BIO4 Biologics. In: Stryker. 2017. Available at: https://footankle.stryker.com/en/products/biologics/bio4. Accessed November 25, 2017.
38. Cellentra Advanced Allograft. In: Zimmer Biomet. 2017. Available at: http://www.zimmerbiomet.com/medical-professionals/spine/product/cellentra.html. Accessed November 25, 2017.
39. Map3 Cellular Allogeneic Bone Graft. In: RTI Surgical. 2017. Available at: http://www.rtix.com/en_us/products/product-implant/map3-cellular-allogeneic-bone-graft. Accessed November 25, 2017.
40. Osteocel Family. In: Nuvasive Biologics. 2017. Available at: https://www.nuvasive.com/procedures/featured-offerings/biologics/. Accessed November 25, 2017.
41. OvationOS Viable Bone Matrix. In: Osiris Therapeutics. 2017. Available at: http://osiris.com/OLD/ovationOS. Accessed November 25, 2017.
42. Trinity Evolution. In: Orthofix. 2017. Available at: http://web.orthofix.com/Products/Pages/Trinity-Evolution.aspx. Accessed November 25, 2017.
43. V92 Cellular Bone Matrix. In: Paragon 28. 2017. Available at: http://www.paragon28.com/products/v92-cellular-bone-matrix/. Accessed November 25, 2017.
44. ViviGen Cellular Bone Matrix. In: DePuy Synthes. 2017. Available at: https://www.depuysynthes.com/hcp/spine/products/qs/vivigen-cellular-bone-matrix. Accessed November 25, 2017.
45. D'Ippolito G, Diabria S, Howard G, et al. Marrow-isolated adult multilineage inducible (MIAMI) cells, a unique population of postnatal young and old human cells with extensive expansion and differentiation potential. J Cell Sci 2004;117:2971–81.

The Role of Placental Membrane Allografts in the Surgical Treatment of Tendinopathies

Joel Ang, DPM, MS*, Chih-Kang David Liou, DPM,
Harry P. Schneider, DPM

KEYWORDS

• Amniotic graft • Placental membrane graft • Tendon repair • Tendinopathy

KEY POINTS

- Surgeons have recently started to implant placental membrane grafts in a variety of surgical procedures.
- When used for tendinopathies, placental membrane grafts may allow for increased angiogenesis and decreased scar tissue formation.
- The scientific literature supports use of placental membranes to reduce inflammation and scarring.
- Although current literature for placental membrane graft use is promising, more high-level clinical trials are required.

INTRODUCTION

Placental membrane grafts have been used in the treatment of lower extremity pathologies for more than a century. The earliest documented use of human placental membrane for treatment of wounds was in 1910 when a general surgeon at John Hopkins Hospital used amniotic grafts to supplement skin transplants.[1] In 1913, amniotic membrane grafts were trialed on burn wounds because their use eliminated the need for a donor site.[2] Subsequently in 1940, an ophthalmologist applied harvested placental membranes to conjunctiva and noted formation of new blood vessels as well as full incorporation of the graft into conjunctival tissue.[3] Despite early studies showing

Disclosure Statement: J. Ang and C-.K.D. Liou have nothing to disclose. H.P. Schneider is a paid consultant for Osiris Therapeutics.
Podiatric Medicine and Surgery, Department of Surgery, Cambridge Health Alliance, Harvard Medical School, 1493 Cambridge Street, Cambridge, MA 02139, USA
* Corresponding author. Department of Surgery, Division of Podiatry, 1493 Cambridge Street, Cambridge, MA 02139.
E-mail address: joelangdpm@gmail.com

Clin Podiatr Med Surg 35 (2018) 311–321
https://doi.org/10.1016/j.cpm.2018.02.004

some benefit with the application of human placental grafts, the increased risk of disease transmission prevented their widespread use. This increased risk was primarily due to the crude methods of harvesting as well as the lack of adequate health screenings for donors. Suboptimal graft harvesting and processing also led to the unintentional removal and destruction of live mesenchymal stem cells, decreasing the efficacy of the graft itself. In the past decade, harvesting, processing, and preservation methods have significantly improved. Placental membrane grafts are now obtained from volunteer donors, all of whom undergo significant screening protocols for hepatitis B and hepatitis C, syphilis, cytomegalovirus, HIV, and tuberculosis.[4] Once the placental membranes are harvested, they undergo a thorough sterilization process prior to preservation. Numerous companies are now manufacturing placental membrane grafts, with a wide variety of product types available for physicians to choose from.

One clarification is required prior to further discussion about grafts. The term, *amniotic graft*, has often been used as a catch-all phrase for any product derived from the placental membrane. This phrase can be confusing for physicians attempting to delineate one product from another. The placental membrane consists of 3 primary layers: the amnion, the chorion, and the uterine decidual tissue.[5] The amnion layer, which in utero is in direct contact with the embryo, is composed of 5 distinct layers: the epithelium, basement membrane, compact layer, fibroblast layer, and intermediate/spongy layer.[6] The chorion layer, which is 3 times to 4 times thicker than the amnion, consists of a cellular layer, a reticular layer, a pseudobasement membrane, and a trophoblast layer.[6] Placental membrane grafts are derived from 1 or both of these 2 layers. There are grafts that contain just the amnion layer and, strictly speaking, only these should be called amniotic grafts. Other products contain just the chorion layer, whereas some contain both the amnion and chorion layer. For the purpose of this article, the term, *placental membrane graft,* is used as an all-encompassing phrase, whereas the term, *amniotic graft,* refers exclusively to products containing just the amnion layer.

The amnion and chorion layers contain multiple growth factors, mesenchymal stem cells, and collagen, which all contribute to the healing process. Specific growth factors found in the grafts include epidermal growth factor, basic fibroblast growth factor, keratinocyte growth factor, vascular endothelial growth factor, transforming growth factor (TGF), nerve growth factor, as well as several other chemokines and cytokines.[6] A majority of these growth factors have been found within the chorion layer.[7] A recent article by Dinh and colleagues[8] provides an excellent overview of each growth factor and its particular role in the healing cycle.

Although research regarding the specific physiologic processes triggered by placental membrane grafts is ongoing, many investigators have noted numerous regenerative benefits of these grafts. First, in vitro and in vivo applications have shown increased native stem cell recruitment.[9,10] Although newer research has shown that mesenchymal stem cells do not themselves differentiate into native host tissue, the mesenchymal stem cells are nevertheless able to attract the host stem cells to the desired area.[11] These host cells then differentiate locally as needed for healing. Second, placental membrane grafts promote angiogenesis. After application of amniotic grafts on chronic wounds, for example, significant new blood vessel formation was noted with both histologic and immunohistologic evaluation.[12] Third, placental membrane grafts are immune privileged and have shown the ability to down-regulate local inflammation. These characteristics are believed secondary to high levels of tissue inhibitor of metalloproteinase, interleukin 10, and interleukin 1RA found in grafts.[13] These cytokines reduce metalloproteinase activity and, therefore, down-regulate the inflammatory phase. This decreased inflammation has 2 touted benefits. By being immune privileged, the placental membrane grafts are able to remain viable for a longer period of time prior to triggering a host foreign body response. This extends the time frame for which the graft growth factors and chemokines can function. By down-regulating local inflammation, there is reduced fibrotic and scar tissue formation, allowing for the generation of a more ideal repair site.

In the modern era, placental membrane grafts have been used primarily in the realm of wound care, aiding the normal healing cascade of hemostasis, inflammation, proliferation, and remodeling. Recently, surgeons are beginning to implant and primarily close over placental membrane grafts to take advantage of the aforementioned benefits. There are specific surgical procedures for which placental membrane grafts would be most beneficial, all of which primarily benefit from improved angiogenesis with decreased inflammation and scar tissue formation. Such procedures would include resection of tarsal coalitions, nerve decompressions, nerve neurolysis, and tendon repairs. Any revisional procedures where scar tissue formation is anticipated can also greatly benefit from the use of a placental membrane graft. The primary goal of this article is to discuss the use of placental membrane grafts for tendinopathies, with a particular focus on rationale, surgical technique, and other important considerations.

RATIONALE

Tendon regeneration occurs through 3 main phases: inflammation, proliferation, and remodeling. During the inflammatory stage, angiogenic factors are secreted and are critical in the formation of vascular tissue at the site of injury.[14] Fibroblasts are also recruited, contributing to healing by producing collagen type III.[14] Placental membrane grafts are a natural aid in this first stage of regeneration, theoretically increasing both angiogenesis and the recruitment of fibroblasts. The proliferative phase occurs several days later, which primarily consists of proteoglycan and collagen formation. This is when fibroblasts are at their peak activity level and potentially when placental membrane grafts are most beneficial. Studies have demonstrated acute elevation of TGF-β—a cytokine produced by fibroblasts—after tendon injuries.[15,16] This elevation has been implicated as a prime contributor of scarring and fibrosis during healing. If the elevation of TGF-β can be controlled, then scarring can be reduced. One study examined 2 sets of transected tendons in vivo, with a control group compared against a group of tendons treated with TGF-β antibodies.[17] Flexor tendons treated with TGF-β antibodies showed a significant reduction in collagen type I and scar tissue production in comparison to control tendons. Treated tendons also showed significant differences in range of motion at 4 weeks and 8 weeks postoperatively.[17] Although placental membranes do not contain TGF-β antibodies, they do contain hyaluronic acid, which has been shown to inhibit TGF-β.[4] Similar antiscarring properties, therefore, may be obtained with use of placental membrane grafts. Additionally, numerous animal studies have shown an increase in both the percentage of collagen type III within the tendon and the overall tendon strength after placental membrane graft application.[18,19] Although the exact biochemical pathways by which grafts allow for an increased collagen percentage have not been determined, there is a growing body of evidence to suggest that placental membrane grafts do provide beneficial outcomes.

Care should be taken, however, not to use placental membrane grafts as a structural support product. Placental membrane grafts do contain multiple types of collagen and are able to withstand some forces, but they should not be used to augment weaker constructs.[20] In cases where some gaping remains after primary repair, for example, a more robust product with a greater collagen composition is indicated. Alternatively, a tendon transfer or an allograft tendon may be used. Simply put, a placental membrane graft may assist in strengthening a tendon over time but should never be the primary strengthener in prevention of reruptures. The final remodeling phase occurs 4 weeks to 6 weeks after injury, a time period by which placental membrane grafts have been fully degraded. Grafts, therefore, are not believed to directly affect the remodeling process of tendons.

Naturally, even without placental membrane grafts, the body has the ability to heal tendons on its own. After the appropriate surgical procedure, a majority of patients with tendinous injuries are likely to progress to uneventful healing. For patients who are evaluated to have tendon pathologies secondary to excessive scar tissue formation, however, or for patients undergoing revisional surgery, placental membrane grafts enter the fold as a tool to assist in obtaining desirable surgical outcomes. Two surgical case examples in which placental membrane grafts were used at the site of injury are discussed.

CASE 1

A healthy 29-year-old male patient presented to the clinic with chronic left lateral rearfoot and ankle pain. MRI examination of the left ankle indicated a split tear of the peroneus brevis tendon with a low-lying muscle belly. The patient underwent an initial surgery of the left ankle with resection of the low-lying muscle belly and retubularization of the tendon without complications. Unfortunately, the patient continued to experience pain at the lateral ankle, specifically at the site of the peroneus brevis repair in the postoperative period. There was also decreased eversion of the subtalar joint noted during clinical examination. An updated MRI, obtained approximately 8 months after the initial surgery, demonstrated residual inflammation at the repair site. Therefore, a decision was made to take the patient back to the operating room for resection of scar tissue with the application of an amniotic graft.

Intraoperatively, there was notable fibrosis of the surrounding soft tissue. Once incision was made through the peroneal tendon sheath, there was appreciable synovitis and scarring of the peroneal tendons. After debulking of the peroneal tendons, the tendons were carefully examined and noted to be free of any structural tears. An amniotic graft was placed between the peroneal tendons, just posterior to the lateral malleolus, because this was the site of maximal adhesion (**Fig. 1**). The surrounding peroneal

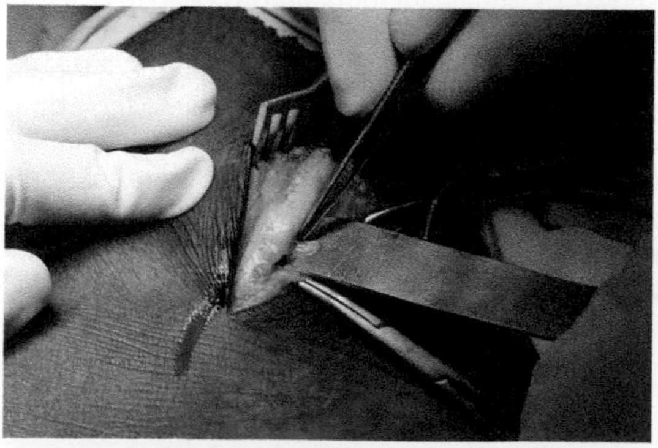

Fig. 1. Amniotic graft placed between the peroneal tendons, just posterior to the lateral malleolus, at the site of maximal adhesion.

tendon sheath was then closed with absorbable suture. The remaining subcutaneous and skin structures were then closed in a standard fashion.

Postoperatively, the patient was made non–weight-bearing for 4 weeks in an immobilization boot. Physical therapy was initiated at the 4-week mark, and the patient returned to full activity 2 months after surgery without pain. Two years later, the patient returned to clinic with some minor discomfort over the peroneal tendons. After receiving 2 corticosteroid injections and undergoing additional physical therapy, the patient was noted to have full resolution of his prior symptoms.

CASE 2

A 33-year-old woman presented to clinic with chronic left Achilles tendon pain, with no relief from a host of conservative treatments, including physical therapy and immobilization. On the patient's initial physical examination, she was noted to have appropriate muscle strength without obvious tendon defect. There was tenderness to palpation appreciated at the posterior aspect of the calcaneus, at the insertion of the Achilles. Radiograph evaluation revealed a retrocalcaneal exostosis, whereas MRI evaluation revealed hypertrophy of the Achilles tendon with partial tears at the level of the retrocalcaneal exostosis. The patient underwent a detachment and reattachment repair of the Achilles, with excision of the retrocalcaneal exostosis. She also underwent a Strayer gastrocnemius recession due to concomitant equinus.

Unfortunately, 2 weeks after surgery the patient experienced a fall, although no palpable defects were appreciated on clinical examination. As she transitioned to weight bearing in a controlled ankle motion boot, she experienced pain with ambulation and focal tenderness to palpation at the watershed region of the Achilles tendon. The area of tenderness was proximal to the site of initial repair. Updated MRI was suggestive of a partial thickness tear at the medial aspect of the tendon. With no resolution of pain despite the continued use of a controlled ankle motion boot, the patient was brought back to the operating room 6 months after her initial surgery for an additional repair of the Achilles tendon.

Intraoperatively, a bulbous appearance of the Achilles tendon was noted secondary to scar tissue. Once the hypertrophied areas were resected, partial tears were appreciated at the medial and central aspects of the watershed region. The tendon was deemed robust enough and did not required additional end to end repair. In an attempt to prevent additional scar formation, half of a placental membrane graft was placed within the Achilles tendon (**Fig. 2**). The graft was secured proximal and distal to the partial tears with absorbable suture. After closure of the peritenon, the remaining half of the placental membrane graft was applied and secured in place with absorbable suture to reduce the risk of wound dehiscence (**Fig. 3**). The remaining subcutaneous and skin structures were then closed in a standard fashion.

Postoperatively, the patient remained non–weight-bearing for 4 weeks prior to transitioning to weight bearing as tolerated in an immobilization boot. With physical therapy, the patient's swelling and tenderness to the Achilles tendon resolved. Two months after the second surgery, she endorsed pain-free ambulation in a regular sneaker.

TECHNICAL CONSIDERATIONS

There are various forms of placental membrane graft available in the market, ranging from dehydrated products to cryopreserved live tissue to injectable amniotic fluid. Dehydrated grafts are classified into either a membrane or micronized form by virtue of the processing technique. Membrane grafts are formed by dehydration of the

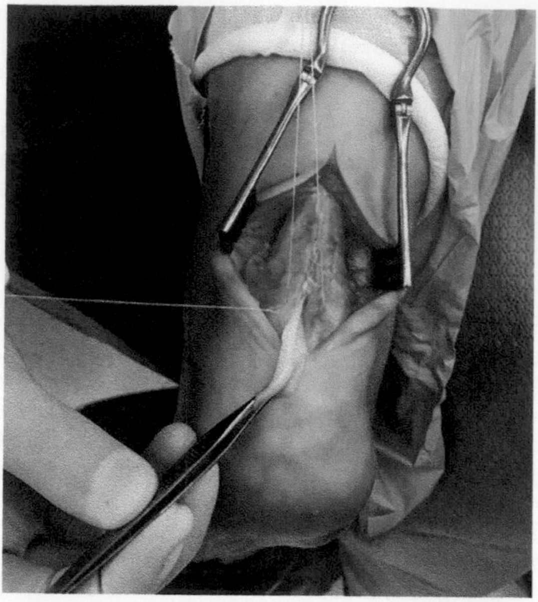

Fig. 2. Half of a placental membrane graft was placed within the Achilles tendon to prevent additional scar formation.

placental membrane in a controlled manner, which removes moisture and cell viability. Micronized grafts are formed by passing the graft through 180-μm and 25-μm filters, sieving for particulate sizing, transforming the amniotic layer into an injectable fluid.[21] Cryopreserved grafts, on the other hand, retain a structure more akin to their in vivo state. Cryopreserved amniotic and amnion/chorion grafts are relatively thin, with a

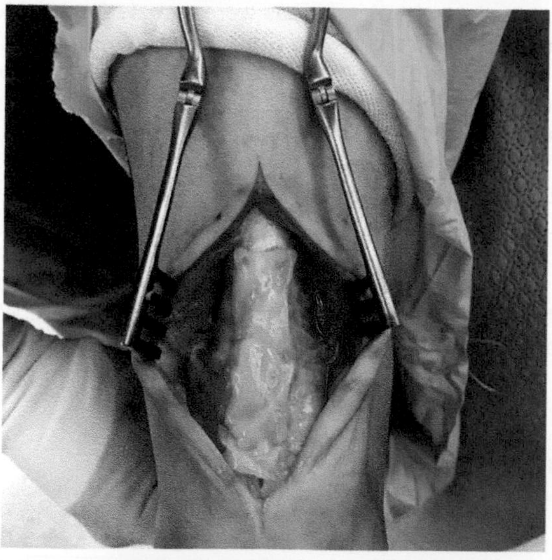

Fig. 3. Remaining half of the placental membrane graft was applied and secured in place with absorbable suture to reduce the risk of wound dehiscence.

mucus-like consistency that may be challenging to handle. There are also cryopreserved umbilical grafts, which are 10 times thicker than amniotic grafts and are easier to suture in place. Although using injectable amniotic fluid for tendon repairs is theoretically sound, it is challenging to ensure the graft remains at the desired site. As a result, membrane grafts and cryopreserved grafts are generally used in the context of tendon repairs. There are several ways to apply these grafts to a tendon. The method used should be dependent on the desired outcome of the surgery.

The easiest method for graft application is to lay the graft over the site of desired repair. Dehydrated membrane grafts, as well as cryopreserved amniotic and chorionic graft products, are often not robust enough to allow for suture fixation. In general, they are simply applied to the surgical site. Dehydrated grafts are initially rigid in form, allowing for relatively easy handling. Once reconstituted with liquid, however, they can be more challenging to maneuver but easily remain at the site of application. Cryopreserved amniotic and chorionic grafts are more difficult to handle. Thicker umbilical cord grafts may be sutured in place, but as few sutures as possible should be used. The use of excessive suture places an increased demand on the body to break down the foreign material, possibly counteracting the benefits of decreased inflammation and scar tissue formation that the graft provides. One variation for graft application is to circumferentially wrap a graft around the tendon sheath. If there is inadequate tendon sheath present for closure, another possibility is to use the graft itself as the tendon sheath substitute. These 2 circumferential methods can reduce the likelihood of tendon entrapment within extratendinous scar tissue.

For both presented surgical cases, the reduction of scarring between 2 tendons or a tendon sheath and its surrounding structures was desired. In the first case, smooth gliding of the peroneal tendons was required for an optimal outcome. As a result, the amniotic graft was applied in between the peroneal tendons at the area of maximal adhesion. An amniotic graft was chosen for this procedure because an amnion/chorion or umbilical graft would have been too thick to apply between the tendons. No sutures were required for positioning because the graft was closed within the peroneal tendon sheath. In the second case, motion of both the Achilles tendon within the peritenon and the entire Achilles complex within the surrounding soft tissue was paramount, and therefore a graft was used in 2 separate layers. Additionally, skin integrity is always a concern for revisional open Achilles repairs, and therefore the superficial graft also served to promote incisional wound healing.

DISCUSSION

Historically, placental membrane grafts have been used in the realm of wound care. There has also been extensive documentation of amniotic graft use in the realm of ophthalmology.[20,22] More recently, surgeons from various specialties have begun using placental membrane grafts for other pathologies, including plantar fasciitis, anterior cruciate ligament reconstructions, rotator cuff repairs, nerve decompressions, and even periodontal surgery. To date, placental membrane grafts have provided surgical benefits with virtually no reports of adverse events.

In a case series consisting of 7 patients, open common peroneal nerve decompression was performed with implantation of an amniotic graft.[23] All 7 patients previously underwent failed surgeries, with continual neuropraxia symptoms. The etiologies of initial neuropraxia ranged from total knee arthroplasty to high-grade ankle sprains to direct trauma. The amniotic graft served to decrease adhesion and inflammation and to assist in nerve regeneration. Common peroneal nerve decompressions were performed with circumferential epineurotomy as well as internal and external neurolysis. Subsequently, nerve fascicles were wrapped with an amniotic graft and a collagen nerve conduit. Seven months postoperatively, 5 of the 7 patients showed full recovery of nerve function as measured by motor strength, range of motion, and nerve conduction velocities. The remaining 2 patients achieved partial recovery. Sixteen months postoperatively, all 7 patients showed no recurrence of prior symptoms.[23]

Amniotic grafts have also been used as interpositional material after tarsal coalition resections. In a study involving 14 patients, amniotic grafts were used in combination with umbilical cords after resection of 7 calcaneonavicular coalitions and 7 talonavicular coalitions.[24] With an average follow-up period of 19 months, no postoperative complications were noted. Patients noted a significant improvement in pain postoperatively, with 64% of patients evaluated to have an increase in range of motion. Although 29% of patients were found to have recurrence of the coalition on CT scan, the investigators concluded that this recurrence rate was comparable to that of interposition with fat, the extensor digitorum brevis muscle, or bone wax.[24]

Current advancements in graft harvesting, processing, and preservation mean that a high number of mesenchymal stem cells remain viable within certain placental membrane grafts. This has shown to be true even after completion of graft thaw cycles.[25] One major concern with implantation of cryopreserved placental grafts is the presence of these live stem cells. Theoretically, stem cells are able to proliferate independently, raising worry for cancer development. It is important, however, to distinguish between 2 major stem cell types—the embryonic stem cell and the mesenchymal stem cell. Embryonic stem cells are isolated from the inner mass of blastocysts and have the potential to form into any cell type. In animal model studies, teratoma formations have been discovered after injection of embryonic stem cells.[26] To date, controlling differentiation of embryonic stem cells has proved an extremely challenging task. As a result, they have not been widely used despite their vast theoretic potential. Mesenchymal stem cells, on the other hand, are mature stem cells that are multipotent and lineage restricted. They are found in a variety of adult tissue types. Placental membrane grafts contain only mesenchymal stem cells. To date, teratoma formation and tumorigenicity after injection of mesenchymal stem cells into either animal or human patients have not been reported.

To further confirm nontumorigenicity of mesenchymal stem cells, Ruan and colleagues[27] isolated mesenchymal stem cells and performed a karyotype analysis. In this study, mesenchymal stem cells were exposed to colchicine, a process that terminated the cells at different stages of proliferation. The stem cells were then cured and examined under the microscope, with specific focus on individual cell chromosomes. Any irregular replication or abnormal division of chromosomes during the mitotic phase was noted as chromosomal alteration. The mesenchymal cells were analyzed at different passages of mitosis, and no spontaneous chromosomal alterations were noted. The authors subsequently concluded that mesenchymal stem cells do not have tumorigenic potential.[27] Phermthai and colleagues[28] were also able to demonstrate the similar chromosomal stability by karyotype analysis.

Recent research suggests mesenchymal stem cells may have some antitumor potential. Ayuzawa and colleagues[29] obtained umbilical cord derived mesenchymal stem cells and examined their effects on mice transplanted with human breast carcinoma MDA 231 cells. These cells were chosen specifically for their ability to metastasize to the lung. The mice were randomized into 2 groups, with 1 group receiving 3 injections of saline and the other group receiving 3 injections of human umbilical stem cells. Thirty days after inoculation with tumor cells, the mice were sacrificed and lung tissue samples were thoroughly analyzed. In mice that received mesenchymal stem cells injections, significant attenuation of tumor growth in the lung was appreciated.[29] Fascinatingly, immunohistochemical stains showed stem cells adjacent to or within tumor cells but not normal tissue, suggesting tumor targeting by mesenchymal cells. A similar animal study also showed inhibition of a different breast cancer cell, MCF-7, after treatment with human fetus–derived mesenchymal stem cells.[30] The exact antitumorigenic pathway is to be determined, but cytokines, such as tumor necrosis factor-α, TGF-β, and interferon-β, are believed to play a role in inducing tumor cell death.[29,31]

Skeptics of placental membrane grafts rightly point out the lack of solid clinical evidence regarding graft implantation. Although there are countless studies detailing amniotic graft use in the realm of wound care and ophthalmology, the same cannot be said of placental graft use in other applications. For the most part, clinical evidence has been limited to in vitro studies or analyses involving mice, chickens, and horses. The evidence has been promising, but strong scientific literature in human subjects is nonexistent. Only a few human case series exist, as discussed previously. One additional case study does show promising histologic changes 8 months after amniotic graft implantation in a rotator cuff repair.[32] These case studies, however, are not enough to fulfill the burden of proof.

In an attempt to add to the body of scientific evidence, a currently unpublished retrospective review of surgical cases with implantable grafts was performed by the authors of this article at Cambridge Health Alliance in 2017. The inclusion criteria were deep implantation of a placental membrane graft with live viable stem cells and a follow-up period of greater than 12 months. Patients requiring grafts for wound care were excluded from the review. The goal of the review was to evaluate for any postoperative complications secondary to placental membrane graft use. To date, a total of 10 patients have met the inclusion criteria, undergoing a variety of procedures ranging from tendon repairs to subtalar coalition resections to tarsal tunnel decompressions. Only 1 patient had a notable postoperative complication. This patient underwent a wide excision of multiple plantar fibromas on the left foot. One fibroma was grossly embedded in the central band of the plantar fascia, measuring greater than 4 cm in diameter. An amniotic graft was sutured to the central band of the fascia after fibroma excision. Postoperatively, the patient experienced mild cellulitis and a small central wound dehiscence, which resolved with oral antibiotics and local wound care. Although the postoperative complication may have been related to graft implantation, the more likely cause was the extensive soft tissue dissection required to excise multiple plantar fibromas. Therefore, from this small retrospective review, no direct complications from implantation of placental membrane grafts were noted.

In summary, placental membrane grafts are a remarkable tool for any foot and ankle surgeon. They have the potential to decrease inflammation and scarring while increasing angiogenesis and collagen deposition, which are all important factors when addressing tendinopathies. Although there is an increasing body of evidence to suggest the benefits placental membrane grafts as an implantable material, more research is required to fully justify their consistent use.

REFERENCES

1. Davis JS. Skin transplantation. Johns Hopkins Hospital Reports 1910;15:307–96.
2. Stern M. The grafting of preserved amniotic membrane to burned and ulcerated surfaces, substituting skin grafts: a preliminary report. JAMA 1913;60(13):973–4.
3. De Rotth A. Plastic repair of conjunctival defects with fetal membranes. Arch Ophthalmol 1940;23(3):522–5.

4. Koizumi NJ, Inatomi TJ, Sotozono CJ, et al. Growth factor mRNA and protein in preserved human amniotic membrane. Curr Eye Res 2000;20(3):173–7.
5. Strauss JF. Extracellular matrix dynamics and fetal membrane rupture. Reprod Sci 2013;20(2):140–53.
6. Zelen CM, Snyder RJ, Serena TE, et al. The use of human amnion/chorion membrane in the clinical setting for lower extremity repair: a review. Clin Podiatr Med Surg 2015;32(1):135–46.
7. Koob TJ, Lim JJ, Zabek N, et al. Cytokines in single layer amnion allografts compared to multilayer amnion/chorion allografts for wound healing. J Biomed Mater Res B Appl Biomater 2015;103(5):1133–40.
8. Dinh T, Braunagel S, Rosenblum BI. Growth factors in wound healing: the present and the future? Clin Podiatr Med Surg 2015;32(1):109–19.
9. Koob TJ, Rennert R, Zabek N, et al. Biological properties of dehydrated human amnion/chorion composite graft: implications for chronic wound healing. Int Wound J 2013;10(5):493–500.
10. Koob TJ, Lim JJ, Massee M, et al. Angiogenic properties of dehydrated human amnion/chorion allografts: therapeutic potential for soft tissue repair and regeneration. Vasc Cell 2014;6:10.
11. Koob TJ, Lim JJ, Massee M, et al. Properties of dehydrated human amnion/chorion composite grafts: implications for wound repair and soft tissue regeneration. J Biomed Mater Res B Appl Biomater 2014;102(6):1353–62.
12. Faulk WP, Matthews R, Stevens PJ, et al. Human amnion as an adjunct in wound healing. Lancet 1980;1(8179):1156–8.
13. Insausti CL, Blanquer M, García-hernández AM, et al. Amniotic membrane-derived stem cells: immunomodulatory properties and potential clinical application. Stem Cells Cloning 2014;7:53–63.
14. Docheva D, Müller SA, Majewski M, et al. Biologics for tendon repair. Adv Drug Deliv Rev 2015;84:222–39.
15. Ngo M, Pham H, Longaker MT, et al. Differential expression of transforming growth factor-beta receptors in a rabbit zone II flexor tendon wound healing model. Plast Reconstr Surg 2001;108(5):1260–7.
16. Klein MB, Yalamanchi N, Pham H, et al. Flexor tendon healing in vitro: effects of TGF-beta on tendon cell collagen production. J Hand Surg Am 2002;27(4):615–20.
17. Xia C, Yang X, Wang YZ, et al. Tendon healing in vivo and in vitro: neutralizing antibody to TGF-β improves range of motion after flexor tendon repair. Orthopedics 2010;33(11):809.
18. Kueckelhaus M, Philip J, Kamel RA, et al. Sustained release of amnion-derived cellular cytokine solution facilitates achilles tendon healing in rats. Eplasty 2014;14:e29.
19. Philip J, Hackl F, Canseco JA, et al. Amnion-derived multipotent progenitor cells improve achilles tendon repair in rats. Eplasty 2013;13:e31.
20. Malhotra C, Jain AK. Human amniotic membrane transplantation: different modalities of its use in ophthalmology. World J Transplant 2014;4(2):111–21.
21. Lei J, Priddy LB, Lim JJ, et al. Dehydrated human amnion/chorion membrane (DHACM) allografts as a therapy for orthopedic tissue repair. Tech Orthop 2017;32(3):149–57.
22. Rahman I, Said DG, Maharajan VS, et al. Amniotic membrane in ophthalmology: indications and limitations. Eye (Lond) 2009;23(10):1954–61.
23. Rodriguez-collazo E, Tamire Y. Open surgical implantation of a viable cryopreserved placental membrane after decompression and neurolysis of common peroneal nerve: a case series. J Orthop Surg Res 2017;12(1):88.

24. Covell DJ, Cohen B, Ellington JK, et al. The use of cryo-preserved umbilical cord plus amniotic membrane tissues in the resection of tarsal coalition. Foot & Ankle Orthopaedics 2016;1(1).
25. Perepelkin NM, Hayward K, Mokoena T, et al. Cryopreserved amniotic membrane as transplant allograft: viability and post-transplant outcome. Cell Tissue Bank 2016;17(1):39–50.
26. Swijnenburg RJ, Sheikh AY, Robbins RC. Comment on "transplantation of undifferentiated murine embryonic stem cells in the heart: teratoma formation and immune response". FASEB J 2007;21(7):1290.
27. Ruan ZB, Zhu L, Yin YG, et al. Karyotype stability of human umbilical cord-derived mesenchymal stem cells during in vitro culture. Exp Ther Med 2014; 8(5):1508–12.
28. Phermthai T, Odglun Y, Julavijitphong S, et al. A novel method to derive amniotic fluid stem cells for therapeutic purposes. BMC Cell Biol 2010;11:79.
29. Ayuzawa R, Doi C, Rachakatla RS, et al. Naïve human umbilical cord matrix derived stem cells significantly attenuate growth of human breast cancer cells in vitro and in vivo. Cancer Lett 2009;280(1):31–7.
30. Qiao L, Xu ZL, Zhao TJ, et al. Dkk-1 secreted by mesenchymal stem cells inhibits growth of breast cancer cells via depression of Wnt signalling. Cancer Lett 2008; 269(1):67–77.
31. Kang NH, Hwang KA, Kim SU, et al. Potential antitumor therapeutic strategies of human amniotic membrane and amniotic fluid-derived stem cells. Cancer Gene Ther 2012;19(8):517–22.
32. Protzman NM, Stopyra GA, Hoffman JK. Biologically enhanced healing of the human rotator cuff: 8-month postoperative histological evaluation. Orthopedics 2013;36(1):38–41.

Mesenchymal Stem Cell Applications for Joints in the Foot and Ankle

Garrett Melick, DPM[a], Najwah Hayman, DPM[a], Adam S. Landsman, DPM, PhD[b,*]

KEYWORDS

• Mesenchymal stem cells • MSC • Foot joint pain

KEY POINTS

- There are limited options for definitive treatment of degenerative joint disease.
- Mesenchymal stem cells (MSCs) have been utilized for the treatment of other types of chronic musculoskeletal pathology.
- The use of MSCs in foot and ankle joint pathology is currently limited.

INTRODUCTION

Degenerative joint disease presents inherent complexity with treatment because of its progressive nature, and as a result, there are limited options for definitive treatment. Mesenchymal stem cells (MSCs) have been implicated in treatment of such chronic musculoskeletal pathology, but their use in foot and ankle pathology is currently limited because of its relative novel introduction into the foot and ankle literature. This article compiles relevant literature regarding MSC injection for intra-articular pathology of the foot and ankle.

Degenerative changes in the foot and ankle revolve around various types of arthritis. Osteoarthritis frequently occurs in the first metatarsal phalangeal joint and is one of the most commonly attacked joints after the knee. Osteoarthritis also appears in the subtalar, talonavicular, and midtarsal joints. This is further exacerbated by biomechanical abnormalities that add further stress to the joints, such as ankle joint instability that can lead to injury of the joint surface, and cartilaginous degeneration.

Rheumatoid arthritis is characterized by lateral deviation of all five digits at the level of the metatarsal phalangeal joints, similar to the deformity seen in the hand with ulnar

Disclosure: The authors have nothing to disclose.

[a] Cambridge Health Alliance, 1493 Cambridge Street, Cambridge, MA 02139, USA; [b] Division of Podiatric Surgery, Department of Surgery, Cambridge Health Alliance, Harvard Medical School, 1493 Cambridge Street, Floor 2, Cambridge, MA 02139, USA
* Corresponding author.
E-mail address: alandsman@cha.harvard.edu

Clin Podiatr Med Surg 35 (2018) 323–330
https://doi.org/10.1016/j.cpm.2018.02.007 podiatric.theclinics.com
0891-8422/18/

deviation of the metacarpal phalangeal joints. Psoriatic arthritis also attacks the foot, and is noted in the toes and metatarsals. These inflammatory, autoimmune conditions have a markedly different cause than osteoarthritis, but still result in painful range of motion.

In theory, the idea of MSC therapy in the joints of the foot and ankle is to counteract inflammation, and stimulate new cartilage formation. In this review of the literature, the authors analyze the literature available on other joints in the body, and the limited data related specifically to the foot and ankle, to determine what may be gained by MSC injection therapy. The goals of MSC therapy are described in **Box 1**.

There are many types of preparations used to provide MSCs. Autologous cells are captured from various sources including liposuction aspirate or cryopreserved umbilical tissue. In the office setting, most of the time the MSC injections are sourced from donated tissues, particularly amniotic fluid. The contributions of autologous and allogeneic MSCs are significantly different. Most importantly, the biggest distinction is that autologous MSCs may survive long enough to differentiate, and develop into chondrocytes, or whatever other cell line is needed, whereas allogeneic cells cannot survive and integrate into the recipient's body. Instead, they act as a valuable source of cytokines and serve to attract the recipient's own stem cells to the area of injection, before being destroyed by the recipient's immune system. Nonetheless, the authors hope to show that there is substantial value in allogeneic stem cell therapy.

IN VITRO EXPERIENCES WITH MESENCHYMAL STEM CELLS

In vitro studies have shown that MSCs promote chondrocyte proliferation and extracellular matrix element synthesis, specifically aggrecan and type II collagen, both ubiquitous in normal cartilaginous tissue.[1] In addition to promoting the differentiation of chondrocytes and extracellular matrix elements, MSCs also exhibit anti-inflammatory, immunomodulatory, and trophic activities that support the chondral tissue reparative process. Specifically, mesenchymal precursor cells (MPCs) have receptors that bind to and inhibit interleukin-6, tumor necrosis factor-α, interleukin-1, and interleukin-17. This mechanism also acts to increase secretion of prostaglandin E_2 and indoleamine 2,3-dioxygenase, which act to promote an anti-inflammatory T-cell response. *In vitro* studies have also demonstrated that when synovial and cartilaginous tissue are exposed to MSCs, there is reduced expression of matrix metalloproteases, which are known to be potent mediators of cartilage destruction when upregulated and are also strongly associated with inflammatory joint pain.[2]

With all of these beneficial downstream effects in mind, it is important to note that MSCs exhibit an indirect relationship with recipient age, thus leading to decreased migration of endogenous MSCs to sites of intra-articular pathology (**Fig. 1**). Specifically, as we age, there is a dramatic loss of stem cells able to be attracted and

Box 1
Goals of mesenchymal stem cell therapy in the foot and ankle

- Stimulate regrowth of native tissues
- Optimize function of existing tissues
- Reduce pain
- Prevent continued destruction of native tissues
- Reduce or eliminate progression of degenerative disease

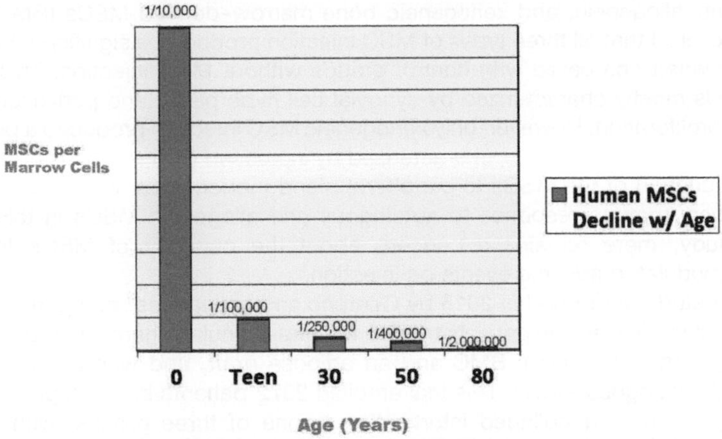

Fig. 1. Incidence of mesenchymal stem cells in adipose tissue decreases with age.

recruited to the site. At birth, 1/10,000 cells are MSCs but by age 50, that figure drops to 1/400,000.

Other interventional strategies have been performed to augment cartilaginous repair. Implantation of chondrocytes and bone marrow concentrate (BMC) have demonstrated promising results for cartilaginous defects. Despite favorable outcomes of chondrocyte implantation for cartilaginous defects, its utility is only indicated for smaller chondral defects. With regard to BMC, it has been acknowledged that the content of MSCs in BMC is actually low at only 0.001% of all mononuclear cells present.[1]

Another benefit of intra-articular injection of MSCs lies in the nature of its biodistribution. Distribution of MSCs is significantly altered when injected intravenously versus intra-articularly, according to results of a recent rabbit model scintigraphy-based study.[1] Intravenously, injected MSCs accumulate to a large extent in the lung parenchyma, whereas intra-articular injected MSCs remain for the most part within the local injection site.[3] By maintaining its prolonged effect within the joint cavity of concern, intra-articular injections thus provide a safe and precise method of intervention for joint pathology.

One area that may need further exploration is the ability of autologous MSCs to adhere to joint surfaces. Optimizing intra-articular MSC adhesion remains a multifactorial process, requiring optimization of adhesion kinetics and removal of local endogenous factors that prevent adherence. The culture expansion process for MSCs may play an important role in this aspect. Specifically, increased time of the MSC culture process has been associated with increased MSC adhesion to articular cartilage *in vitro*. The theory supporting this finding references the change in integrin subtype with time in culture, but this may need to be delineated further in human models. Previous studies have shown that certain enzymes, such as chondroitinase ABC, enhance chondrocyte adhesion to cartilage surfaces by removing proteoglycans that would normally inhibit adherence.[4] Further studies in vivo should be performed to quantify the parameters necessary to achieve optimal articular cartilage adherence.

MESENCHYMAL STEM CELL LINEAGES AND SAFETY

Investigation of MSC injection is divided into studies involving autologous, allogeneic, and xenogeneic MSC products. In an equine study involving intra-articular injection of autologous, allogeneic, and xenogeneic bone marrow–derived MSCs (BM-MSC), it was discovered that all three types of MSC injection produced a significant histologic response when compared with control groups without MSC injection. This cellular response is mostly characterized by synovial cell hyperplasia and perivascular lymphocytic proliferation. However, only xenogeneic MSC injection produced a persistent immune-modulated response, characterized by increased CD4 positive cell presence on reintroduction of the MSCs to peripheral blood mononuclear cells.[5] Despite lack of sustained immune response to autologous and allogeneic MSCs in this equine model study, there remains a concern about the capacity of MSCs to cause immune-modulated adverse events on injection.

Another study performed in 2016 by Centeno and colleagues[6] compared the incidence of adverse events in patients treated for intra-articular, ligament, and/or tendon pathology with BMC alone, BMC and an adipose graft, and with *in vitro* culture-expanded autologous MSCs. This trial enrolled 2372 patients in a prospective treatment registry for a nonblinded intervention in one of three groups, with average follow-up of 2.2 years. Overall, 325 adverse events in 287 patients were reported. However, only 38 of these events were deemed to be definitively related to the procedure, and only 10 of these events were deemed to be definitively caused by the stem cell introduction. The most common adverse events were pain post-procedure (29% of all adverse events) and pain related to degenerative joint disease (DJD) (28%). Serious adverse events to be concerned about include neoplastic, neurologic, and vascular events. There was a significant increase in the incidence of serious adverse events in the culture-expanded autologous MSC group, but this was perceived to be likely caused by the significantly longer follow-up time for the culture-expanded autologous MSC group when compared with the other two groups.

To minimize risks of immune response, research has been performed to test the immunomodular capacity of certain MPC antigens. Use of monoclonal antibodies specific for MPC surface antigens has shown that MPCs bound by STRO-1 and STRO-3 antibodies have the greatest ability to retain their immunophenotype throughout colony formation, meaning that MPCs with these antibodies should provide the least chance for immune response. Additionally, MPCs bound by these antibodies also conveniently have the greatest clonogenicity when compared with other MPC lineages.[2]

PRACTICAL APPLICATION OF MESENCHYMAL STEM CELLS FOR INTRA-ARTICULAR PATHOLOGY

To our knowledge, there is not yet a randomized controlled trial (RCT) for MSC intra-articular injection of the foot and ankle, but several have been performed for the knee. In 2016, Lamo-Espinosa and colleagues[1] performed an RCT comparing two dose regimens of a single intra-articular injection of GMP-produced autologous bone marrow MSC with hyaluronic acid (HA) for patients with knee osteoarthritis. Outcome measures assessed included incidence of complications or adverse events, range of motion, pain and physical function assessment, and imaging criteria. All outcome measures were assessed at baseline and serial follow-up appointments 3, 6, and 12 months postintervention. Interventional groups included a low-dose group (10×10^6 cultured BM-MSCs in 1.5 mL of lactated Ringer solution and 4 mL of HA) and a high-dose group (100×10^6 cultured BM-MSCs in 3-mL lactated Ringer solution and 4 mL HA). Outcome measures were also tested in a control group receiving one injection of 60 mg (4 mL) of HA. No serious adverse events were reported. Increased sagittal plane range of motion was noted in the bone marrow MSC injections group, and this was seen earlier in the treatment process within the high-dose group than the low-dose group. Pain score according to the Visual Analogue Scale was significantly improved in both MSC injection groups relative to the control group with no significant difference between the low- and high-dose regimens. A scoring system compiling pain, stiffness, and physical function assessment was found to be significantly improved in the MSC injection groups relative to the control group. The high-dose regimen group exhibited a more sustained improvement than the low-dose group at 12 months postintervention. With respect to radiograph analysis of joint space, only the high-dose MSC group exhibited no reduction in knee joint space following treatment. However, it is worth noting that despite randomization of groups, those in the low-dose group had a more advanced stage of osteoarthritis than the other groups on average, which could have skewed these results. Additionally, a verified scoring protocol based on number and location of articular lesions, cartilage thickness, signal intensity, and subchondral bone alteration revealed improvement only in the high-dose MSC group. Overall, results support the use of a high dose of 100×10^6 BM-MSCs for subjective and objective improvement of knee osteoarthritis.[1]

Not surprisingly, allogeneic MSCs provide some benefits over autologous implantation, notably lack of donor site morbidity. Also, there is no need to wait for the culture expansion process following aspiration as seen with autologous MSC injection. Another RCT was performed by Wang and colleagues[2] in 2017 to investigate long-term outcomes of allogeneic MSC injection following anterior cruciate ligament reconstruction. Specifically, two groups were compared: 11 subjects receiving 75 million allogeneic MPCs suspended in HA; and six subjects receiving HA injection alone. None of the subjects had evidence of articular cartilage damage at the time of initial presentation. In particular, STRO-3-positive MPCs were provided for this study from an outside company. Because of the proprietary nature of the colony formation, this cell preparation process was unable to be explained fully. However, it was noted that during the culture expansion process, the human-derived MPCs are exposed to fetal bovine serum. To test for possible immunogenic response, the authors of this study tested anti-HLA panel reactive antibodies, antibovine, and antimurine antibodies at regular intervals via flow cytometry. Other outcome measures assessed included knee pain, function, and quality of life assessment, and objective radiograph and MRI criteria. Despite an initial rise in anti-HLA panel reactive antibodies in the MPC treatment group relative to the control, there were no serious adverse events in the treatment group related to the injection. Also, no significant abnormalities in laboratory markers or vital signs were observed in serial follow-up assessments throughout the course of the study. Relative to the control group, those undergoing allogeneic MPC injection had significantly less pain than the control subjects. MPC injection was associated with significantly reduced subchondral bone remodeling and increased tibiofemoral joint space at 2 years postintervention. Also, MPC injection was correlated with a cartilage-preserving trend, although this was not found to be statistically significant.[2]

Although not as heavily documented in literature thus far, the potential applications for MSC intra-articular injection in the foot and ankle are numerous. The prevalence of osteoarthritis in the foot and ankle make it an easy target for MSC application. In two similar studies involving varus ankle osteoarthritis, the application of autologous adipose-derived MSCs at the site of osteochondral lesion along with corrective was retrospectively compared with patients undergoing the surgery alone. In particular, the MSC injections were performed as an adjunct to arthroscopic marrow stimulation and corrective osteotomy (supramalleolar osteotomy[7] or lateralizing calcaneal osteotomy[8]). Clinical improvement in Visual Analogue Scale scores and American

Orthopaedic Foot and Ankle Society ankle-hindfoot scores was significantly increased in the MSC-injected patients over the surgery-only patients. Also, on removal of hardware, gross arthroscopic examination of the lesion demonstrated significant improvement in the lesions themselves according to an established grading system.[7,8] Besides the more prevalent application to osteoarthritis, there is also certainly potential for its use in cases of avascular necrosis (AVN). Especially with regard to talar AVN, the foot and ankle surgeon has few viable options, mostly limited to offloading, bone grafting, core decompression, talectomy, and arthrodesis.

A recent retrospective study by Hernigou and colleagues[9] sought to compare combined core decompression and percutaneous injection of autologous BMC with core decompression alone in 79 cases of post-traumatic talar AVN before talar collapse. Pain, range of motion, activity, the need for assistive devices, the need for additional surgery, radiographic progression of AVN, MRI lesion mapping, and intralesional MSC counts were among the outcome measures assessed. All patients were followed from initial presentation with talar fracture, with all patients in the study having Hawkins type I or II fractures. Hawkins I fractures were managed conservatively with plaster casting, and Hawkins II fractures were managed with open reduction internal fixation with a 5-mm partially threaded cancellous screw. Following diagnosis of AVN, the stage of talar osteonecrosis was classified according to the Ficat and Arlet system modified for the ankle, and the volume of each talar dome lesion was measured as the ratio of the lesion volume to the volume of the talar dome. Between 1985 and 1995, a total of 34 subjects underwent core decompression alone. Of these 34 patients, 14 subjects had aspiration of the osteonecrosis performed arthroscopically at the time of core decompression, to count the number of MSCs at the injury site. Subsequently, between 1995 and 2012, the next 45 talar AVN patients underwent core decompression and simultaneous percutaneous BMC injection of 20 mL at the site of decompression. All subjects included in the study were assessed every 3 months postintervention over the course of the first 2 years and every year following that until 2016, with a total of 11 patients lost to follow-up and an average 17-year follow-up period for other patients. No significant differences in AVN staging or clinical scores were noted between the two groups at the time of initial assessment. BMC injection was associated with significant reduction in pain and joint symptoms compared with lesion size- and AVN stage-matched control subjects. Most importantly, the rate of talar collapse was significantly less in the BMC-injected group than the control group. Also, in those that required arthrodesis secondary to talar collapse, the rate of fusion was significantly better, and the time to radiographic union was significantly shorter in the BMC treatment group compared with control subjects. MRI comparison of the two groups demonstrated a significant increase in volume of repair to the talar lesion in BMC treatment group (6.53 cm^3) compared with control group (2.1 cm^3), on average. With all of these results considered, histologic samples of bone marrow collected at the time of arthrodesis for talar collapse patients in both groups demonstrated significantly increased MSC concentration at the site of repair in the BMC-treated group when compared with the control group. Until this study, core decompression was indicated for Ficat and Arlet stage I and II AVN of the talus. However, results from this study showed improved results with BMC injection for both of these stages in the presence of core decompression.[9]

MESENCHYMAL STEM CELLS AS IMMUNOLOGIC SUPPRESSOR AND ANTI-INFLAMMATORY

In a paper presented by Smith and colleagues,[10] it was pointed out that allogeneic MSCs, although still immunogenic, seem to survive for extended periods of time. It has been suggested that one reason for this is that MSCs seem to suppress natural killer cells, neutrophils, macrophages, and lymphocytes. Because of this unique property, they may be an effective tool in the treatment of systemic inflammatory conditions, such as rheumatoid arthritis. This action is probably the result of elevation of prostaglandin E_2 levels. There have even been studies that demonstrate that this effect with MSCs may help to prevent immune complications following tissue transplantation. They may even be used as a therapy for other inflammatory conditions, such as acute respiratory distress syndrome. In addition to the direct benefits of reducing painful inflammation, the MSCs may be helpful as part of an adjunctive treatment when allogeneic cartilage grafts are performed.

In a study by Vega and colleagues,[11] allogeneic MSCs were given as an intra-articular injection in patients with knee osteoarthritis. Subsequent MRI demonstrated improvements in the cartilage quality. Additionally, patients reported improvement in pain, quality of life, and decreased disability. The perceived improvements were also found in another knee study performed by Vangsness and colleagues,[12] who demonstrated an increase in meniscus volume after an allogeneic MSC injection for patients with osteoarthritis of the knee.

More recently, a study by Maumus and colleagues[13] described allogeneic MSCs as a potential therapy for specific inflammatory autoimmune diseases, such as rheumatoid arthritis. For MSCs to be an effective treatment of these conditions, a combination of growth and differentiation factors must be available to stimulate chondrocyte proliferation. Hybrid implants containing MSC-coated microcarriers may be injected into a joint, where they can be incorporated into cartilaginous defects to produce hyaline cartilage, rather than fibrocartilage. Thus, MSC therapy acts as an anti-inflammatory to prevent continued degeneration of the joint, while also contributing to actual cartilaginous repair.

DISCUSSION

The use of MSCs for treatment of degenerative joint conditions of the foot and ankle, such as osteoarthritis, and inflammatory autoimmune conditions, such as rheumatoid arthritis, has not been studied extensively. However, there is plenty of evidence, *in vivo* and *in vitro*, that indicates that there are probably some substantial benefits for treating these painful, damaged joints with MSCs. The evidence from patients treated with knee pain strongly suggests that allogeneic MSCs help to thicken and restore cartilage. It also helps to reduce pain, and modulate autoimmune inflammatory arthritis.

In our clinical experience, patients with a variety of painful joint conditions in the foot and ankle have experienced great relief following an intra-articular injection of allogeneic MSCs. To date, we have had good success with treatments of chronic pain in Lisfranc joint following contusions, periarticular stress fractures of the metatarsals, and treatment of joint space narrowing related to symptomatic hallux valgus. Other investigators have also reported significant improvement in the ankle.

Based on our review of the literature, it seems that the principal benefits of MSC injections are the anti-inflammatory and immunosuppressive characteristics. It also seems that in some cases, these MSCs may have the ability to stimulate chondrocyte proliferation. Other chemicals, such as HA, are known inhibitors of matrix metalloproteases, but do not seem to have the concomitant immunosuppressive characteristics, and consequently lack the longevity of effect associated with MSCs.

REFERENCES

1. Lamo-Espinosa JM, Mora G, Blanco JF, et al. Intra-articular injection of two different doses of autologous bone marrow mesenchymal stem cells versus hyaluronic acid in the treatment of knee osteoarthritis: multicenter randomized controlled clinical trial (phase I/II). J Transl Med 2016;14(246):1–9.
2. Wang Y, Shimmin A, Ghosh P, et al. Safety, tolerability, clinical, and joint structural outcomes of a single intraarticular injection of allogeneic mesenchymal precursor cells in patients following anterior cruciate ligament reconstruction: a controlled double-blind randomised trial. Arthritis Res Ther 2017;19(180):1–12.
3. Meseguer-Olmo L, Montellano AJ, Martínez T, et al. Intraarticular and intravenous administration of 99MTc-HMPAO-labeled human mesenchymal stem cells (99MTC-AH-MSCS): in vivo imaging and biodistribution. Nucl Med Biol 2017; 46:36–42.
4. Hung BP, Babalola OM, Bonassar LJ. Quantitative characterization of mesenchymal stem cell adhesion to the articular cartilage surface. J Biomed Mater Res A 2013;101(12):3592–8.
5. Pigott JH, Ishihara A, Wellman ML, et al. Investigation of the immune response to autologous, allogeneic, and xenogeneic mesenchymal stem cells after intra-articular injection in horses. Vet Immunol Immunopathol 2013;156(1–2):99–106.
6. Centeno CJ, Al-Sayegh H, Freeman MD, et al. A multi-center analysis of adverse events among two thousand, three hundred and seventy two adult patients undergoing adult autologous stem cell therapy for orthopaedic conditions. Int Orthop 2016;40:1755–65.
7. Kim YS, Lee M, Koh YG. Additional mesenchymal stem cell injection improves the outcomes of marrow stimulation combined with supramalleolar osteotomy in varus ankle osteoarthritis: short-term clinical results with second-look arthroscopic evaluation. J Exp Orthop 2016;3(12):1–10.
8. Kim YS, Koh YG. Injection of mesenchymal stem cells as a supplementary strategy of marrow stimulation improves cartilage regeneration after lateral sliding calcaneal osteotomy for varus ankle osteoarthritis: clinical and second-look arthroscopic results. Arthroscopy 2016;32(5):878–89.
9. Hernigou P, Dubory A, Flouzat Lachaniette CH, et al. Stem cell therapy in early post-traumatic talus osteonecrosis. Int Orthop 2018. [Epub ahead of print].
10. Smith B, Sigal IR, Grande DA. Immunology and cartilage regeneration. Immunol Res 2015;63(1–3):181–6.
11. Vega A, Martín-ferrero MA, Del Canto F, et al. Treatment of knee osteoarthritis with allogeneic bone marrow mesenchymal stem cells: a randomized controlled trial. Transplantation 2015;99:1681–90.
12. Vangsness CT, Farr J, Boyd J, et al. Adult human mesenchymal stem cells delivered via intra-articular injection to the knee following partial medial meniscectomy: a randomized, double-blind, controlled study. J Bone Joint Surg Am 2014;96(2):90–8.
13. Maumus M, Guérit D, Toupet K, et al. Mesenchymal stem cell-based therapies in regenerative medicine: applications in rheumatology. Stem Cell Res Ther 2011; 2(2):14.

Soft Tissue Reconstruction with Artelon for Multiple Foot and Ankle Applications

Russell D. Petranto, DPM[a,*], Megan Lubin, DPM, MS[a], Robert C. Floros, DPM[a], Darelle A. Pfeiffer, DPM[a], Kerianne Spiess, DPM[a], Robin Lenz, DPM[a], Amanda Crowell, DPM[a], Haseeb Ahmad, DPM[c], Sameep Chandrani, DPM[c], Adam S. Landsman, DPM, PhD[b]

KEYWORDS

• Artelon • Achilles tendon • Tendon graft • Tendon rupture • Peroneal tendon rupture • Synthetic tendon graft

KEY POINTS

- Surgical repair of tendons of the foot and ankle is performed utilizing various methods, including, but not limited to, autografts, allografts, and synthetic grafts.
- Artelon soft tissue reconstruction has multiple foot and ankle applications for traumatic and chronic tendon ruptures of the foot and ankle.
- Artelon has been used successfully as a useful alternative for the reinforcement of tendon repairs compared with autografts and allografts.

There are a wide range of approaches when it comes to the surgical repair of Achilles, posterior tibial, and peroneal tendons. The best method of repair, especially when it comes to the Achilles tendon, is often debated. Aside from simple end-to-end repair, there are many different ways to augment Achilles tendon repairs, including lengthening and grafting. Heikkinen and colleagues[1] found that there were no differences between end-to-end tendoachilles repair compared with augmentation utilizing gastrocnemius fascia turn down flap in acute tendon ruptures. Aktas and colleagues[2] also reported that there was no difference in functional outcome between end-to-end Achilles tendon repair and an end-to-end repair with plantaris augmentation in acute tendon ruptures. In chronic/neglected Achilles tendon ruptures, Ofili and colleagues[3] reported that use of allograft compared favorably with alternatives and was an

Disclosure Statement: The authors have nothing to disclose.

[a] Ocean County Foot & Ankle Surgical Associates, P.C., 54 Bey Lea Road, Toms River, NJ 08753, USA; [b] Division of Podiatric Surgery, Department of Surgery, Cambridge Health Alliance, Harvard Medical School, 1493 Cambridge Street, Floor 2, Cambridge, MA 02139, USA; [c] Residency Program, Veterans Administration Hospital, 385 Tremont Avenue, East Orange, NJ 07018-1023, USA
* Corresponding author.
E-mail address: rpetranto@ocfasa.com

Clin Podiatr Med Surg 35 (2018) 331–342
https://doi.org/10.1016/j.cpm.2018.02.008

acceptable approach with good overall outcomes and low risk. Jennings and Sefton[4] reported that use of synthetic graft allows for quicker functional recovery.

Acute peroneal tendon tears can often be primarily repaired.[5] Chronic peroneal tendon injuries require more extensive treatment options including autologous tendon transfers, tendon lengthening, tenodesis, and the use of allograft, autografts, and synthetic grafts. Mook and Nunley[6] reported that allograft reconstruction can improve strength and decrease pain while maintaining satisfactory patient outcomes. Therefore, allografts are a safe and reasonable alternative in treatment of otherwise irreparable peroneal tendon ruptures. Although a small study, Rapley and colleagues[7] reported that a decellularized dermal matrix provided effective augmentation in repairing chronic degenerated peroneal tendon tears.

Posterior tibialis (PT) tendon ruptures can result from microtrauma due to posterior tibial tendon dysfunction (PTTD), which leads to edema, hemorrhage, scarring, and subsequent weakening of the posterior tibialis tendon.[8] There are various surgical procedures and techniques along with concomitant soft tissue/osseous procedures to correct a flatfoot deformity. PT tendon rupture repairs include tenosynovectomy, primary repair, and augmentation such as flexor digitorum longus (FDL) tenodesis, Cobb procedure, and peroneus brevis tendon transfer.[9] Numerous forms of FDL tendon implantation have been described, including securing the tendon to the periosteum of the navicular or medial cuneiform with nonabsorbable sutures[10] or utilizing bone anchors in the navicular or sustentaculum tali.[11] Gazdag and Cracchiolo[12] advocate spring ligament repair as well, citing it as a necessity to strengthen the static support of the hindfoot. However, it is inconclusive if spring ligament repair results in an overall better outcome. Janis and colleagues[13] found that in 17 cases, 92% of patients were able to return to previous activities with pain relief and ability to walk ranging from fair to excellent following a Cobb procedure. Helal[14] reported better results with the Cobb procedure versus other augmentation procedures including FDL transfers. To the authors' knowledge, there has been no reported studies of usage of synthetic grafts in the correction of acute or chronic PT tendon ruptures.

For over 100 years, different biomaterials have been utilized for augmentation of soft tissue repairs, with the goal of providing additional mechanical strength during the acute healing phase while permitting anatomic mechanical loading and remodeling into organized, functional tissue. Autograft and allografts currently remain the gold standard; however, a disadvantage of these grafts is rapid loss of strength and elasticity due to tissue necrosis and resorption.[15] During remodeling, these avascular grafts are eliminated through phagocytosis, followed by revascularization, cellular infiltration, and matrix remodeling via collagen 1 production to restore mechanical strength and elasticity. This process takes about 12 months to reach maturation and restored functional capacity.[16]

Reinforcement devices made from xenografts, polytetrafluoroethylene (PTFE), polyethylene terephthalate, polypropylene, polyethylene, and carbon fibers have all been used clinically and subsequently abandoned because of poor mechanical properties and device failure. Degradable polydioxanone (PDS) devices were also used and abandoned because of high stiffness, stress shielding, and repair failure.[17–22]

PCL-based polyurethane urea (PUUR) has many desirable qualities for soft tissue reinforcement. It is inert, and less reactive than common biomaterials such as titanium and polystyrene.[23] It is strong and creep-resistant to protect the repair during acute healing; however, it is also hyperelastic to permit loading and stimulation of the tissues during late remodeling.[24,25] It integrates into the repair site without foreign body reaction or phagocytosis, maintains its strength for 4 to 6 years, and is eliminated benignly through hydrolytic degradation.[26]

Artelon (Artelon, Marietta Georgia) is made from extruded and wet-spun fibers of PUUR that have been knitted into textile patches and strips for optimal mechanical properties and ease of use. This material has been studied extensively for various soft tissue reinforcement applications.

Peterson[27] reported on Artelon for anterior cruciate ligament (ACL) reconstruction in a long-term multicenter randomized controlled trial with over 200 patients and 12 years of follow-up. Patients tolerated the Artelon implant well, and demonstrated improved rotational stability (pivot-shift test) versus the control group. Biopsy and histology from 1 to 6 years postoperatively demonstrated excellent integration of the Artelon implant and creeping substitution of ligament regeneration.

CASE 1

A 73-year-old man presented to the office several weeks after slipping and falling in the shower. He reported a dull, aching pain in his right posterior heel.

The patient's past medical history was significant for type 2 diabetes, gout, glaucoma, cataracts, prostate cancer, hyperlipidemia, and morbid obesity (body mass index [BMI] 50.1). On clinical examination, there was no palpable defect to the Achilles tendon. However, there was a palpable mass present proximal to the Achilles insertion, suggesting that a portion of the tendon had recoiled proximally. An MRI was obtained, which revealed moderate-to-severe tendinosis of the distal attachment of the Achilles tendon with a partial tear medially. Recommendation was surgical repair of the Achilles tendon with the Artelon implant.

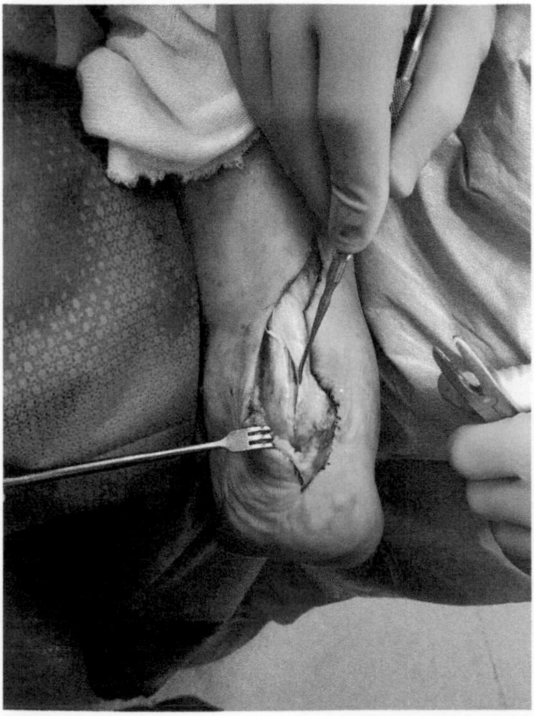

Fig. 1. The Achilles tendon was incised centrally and resected from the calcaneus preserving the most medial and lateral attachments.

The procedure was performed in a prone position with spinal anesthesia and a femoral nerve block. The Achilles tendon was incised centrally and resected from the calcaneus, preserving the most medial and lateral attachments (**Fig. 1**). The medial partial tear was identified, and a significant amount of gouty tophi was resected. A calcaneal spur was also identified and resected (**Fig. 2**). Two bone anchors were inserted into the calcaneus, inferior to the Achilles insertion. The Artelon implant (0.7 cm × 16 cm) was then woven through the Achilles tendon (**Fig. 3**). The anchors were sutured to both the Artelon and the Achilles tendon, with the foot held in neutral position (**Fig. 4**). The tendon was further reinforced with suture, and the paratenon was repaired. The patient was placed in a well-padded below-knee fiberglass cast. He was later discharged to an assisted living facility and received heparin for deep vein thrombosis (DVT) prophylaxis. At 5 weeks postoperatively, he was transitioned into a controlled ankle movement (CAM) boot to begin weight bearing. By 8 weeks postoperatively, the patient had returned to full weight bearing and was living at home. Overall the patient had an excellent outcome with rapid return to function.

CASE 2

A 79-year-old woman presented to the office with right ankle pain and swelling after driving for 6 hours 2 to 3 weeks prior to presentation.

Her medical history was significant for hyperlipidemia and thyroid disorder. On physical examination, she demonstrated pain on palpation along the course of

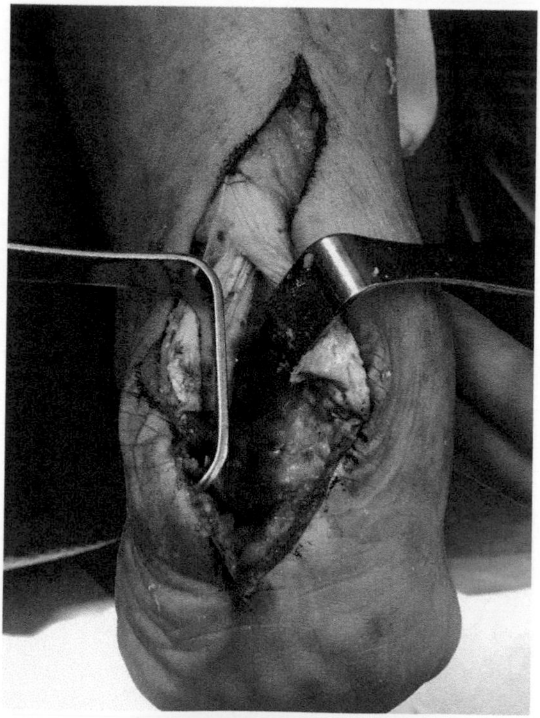

Fig. 2. The medial partial tear was identified and a significant amount of gouty tophi were resected. A calcaneal spur was also identified and resected.

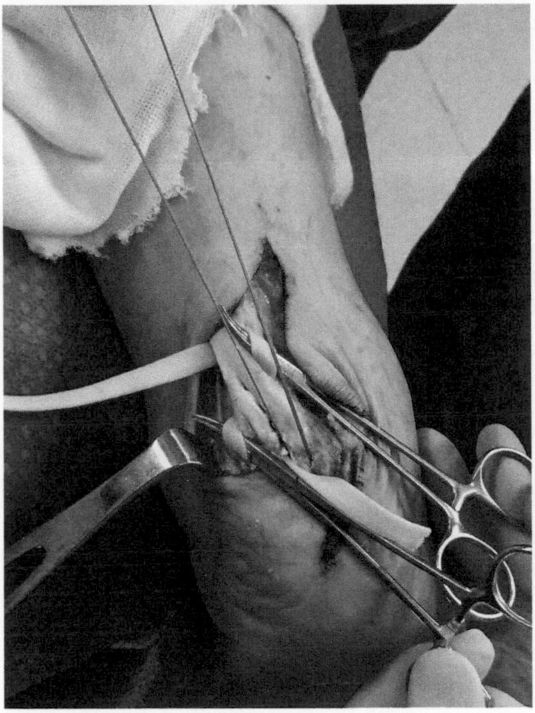

Fig. 3. Two bone anchors were inserted into the calcaneus, inferior to the Achilles insertion. The Artelon implant (0.7 cm × 16 cm) was then woven through the Achilles tendon. (*Courtesy of* Artelon, Marietta, GA.)

the posterior tibial tendon as well as inability to perform a single heel raise on the right foot. She was treated conservatively for 2 months with fiberglass cast and CAM boot immobilization, supportive tapings, and injections of the posterior tibial tendon sheath. Because of the presence of surgical hardware from a prior ankle

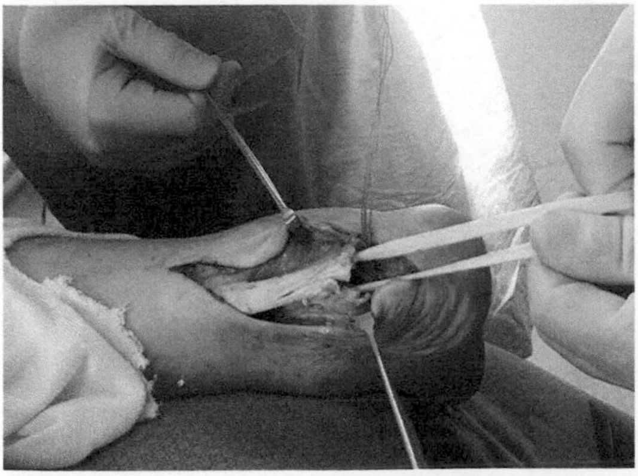

Fig. 4. The anchors were sutured to both the Artelon and the Achilles tendon with the foot held in neutral position. (*Courtesy of* Artelon, Marietta, GA.)

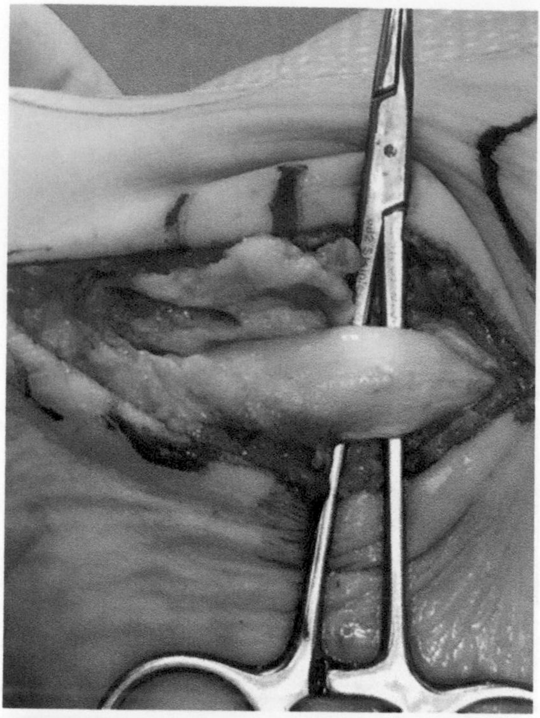

Fig. 5. A complete rupture of the plantar calcaneonavicular spring ligament.

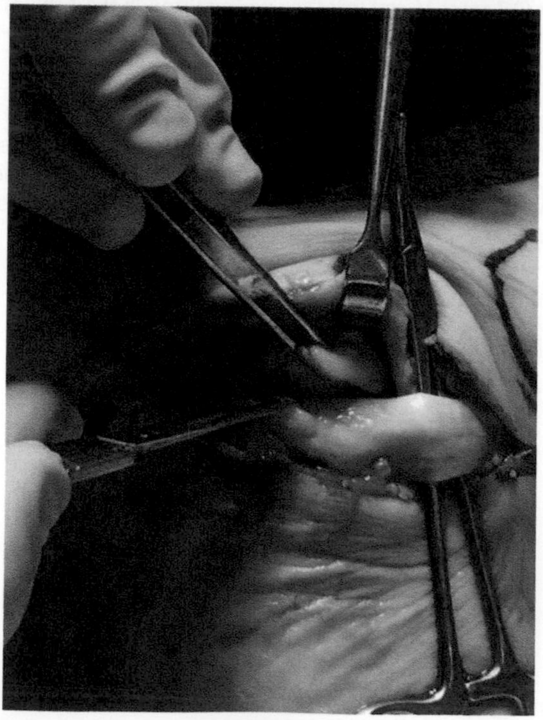

Fig. 6. A longitudinal tear of the posterior tibial tendon.

fracture, an MRI was not obtained. Radiographs demonstrated an enlarged navicular tuberosity but no fractures. The decision was made to proceed with surgical intervention.

The procedure was performed in a supine position under general anesthesia. Because of patient discomfort, the fibular plate was removed first via a standard lateral approach. Next, a curvilinear incision was made extending from posterior to the medial malleolus to the navicular tuberosity. A complete rupture of the plantar calcaneonavicular spring ligament and a longitudinal tear of the posterior tibial tendon were identified (**Figs. 5** and **6**).

The spring ligament was repaired by passing an Artelon strip (0.5 cm × 16 cm) through a drill hole in the navicular and suturing it to the proximal and distal remnants of the ligament. Next, the posterior tibial tendon was incised and debrided from proximal-posterior to distal-anterior, and the Artelon strip was woven through the severed end of the tendon (**Figs. 7** and **8**).

The tendon was further tubularized (**Fig. 9**). The patient was placed in a fiberglass below-knee cast for 6 weeks following surgery and then transitioned into a pneumatic CAM boot and allowed to begin weight bearing. She began physical therapy 2 months postoperatively for strengthening and range of motion. By 3 months postoperatively she reported increased mobility with her right ankle, and by 4 months postoperatively she had returned to baseline with the ability to perform all activities of daily living without the need of an assistive device.

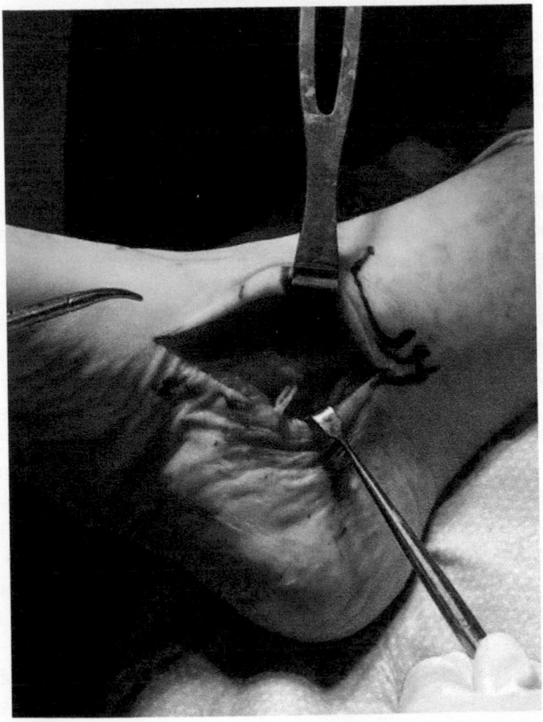

Fig. 7. The spring ligament was repaired by passing an Artelon strip (0.5 cm × 16 cm) through a drill hole in the navicular and suturing it to the proximal and distal remnants of the ligament. (*Courtesy of* Artelon, Marietta, GA.)

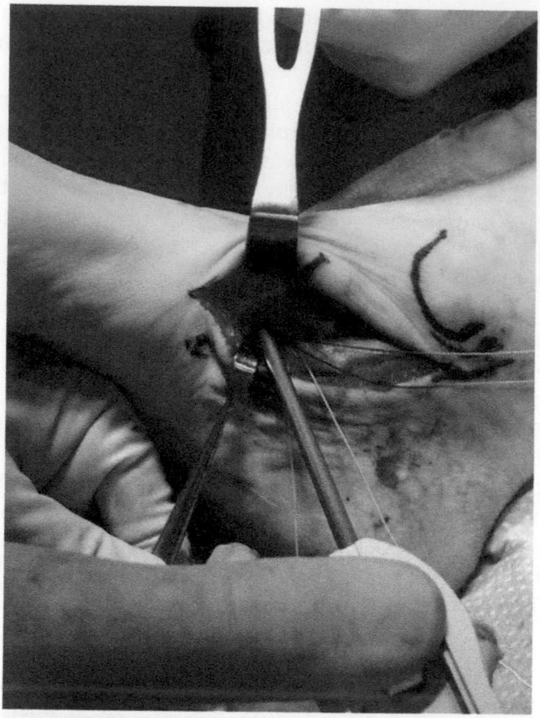

Fig. 8. Next, the posterior tibial tendon was incised and debrided from proximal-posterior to distal-anterior, and the Artelon strip was woven through the severed end of the tendon. (*Courtesy of* Artelon, Marietta, GA.)

CASE 3

A 38-year-old man was seen in the office complaining of sharp left lateral ankle pain. The patient related a history of rolling his left ankle on multiple occasions but was unaware of any recent injury to the ankle. The patient also described the feeling of the ankle giving out often.

His medical history was significant for hypertension, hypercholesterolemia, kidney stones, obesity, gout, and asthma, and surgical history was significant for right wrist ligament repair. On physical examination, there was tenderness with palpation along the course of the peroneal tendon distal to the ankle and at the area of the anterior talofibular ligament and calcaneofibular ligament. Treatment was initiated and included physical therapy, use of an ankle stabilizer, nonsteroidal anti-inflammatory drugs (NSAIDs); rest, ice, compression, and elevation (RICE); and use of orthoses. After 3 weeks a follow-up appointment revealed worsening pain at the lateral ankle, and MRI was recommended at that visit. MRI revealed a partial tear of the peroneus longus and peroneus brevis with tenosynovitis. In addition, there was flattening of the peroneus brevis and attenuation of the anterior talofibular ligament. Six weeks after initiating treatment with no improvement, surgery was planned.

Under general anesthesia, the patient was placed in a lateral decubitus position, and a lateral incision was made along the anatomic course of the peroneal tendons. Dissection revealed a split-thickness tear and tenosynovitis of the peroneus brevis tendon and thickening, tenosynovitis, and an interstitial tear of the peroneus longus tendon (**Fig. 10**).

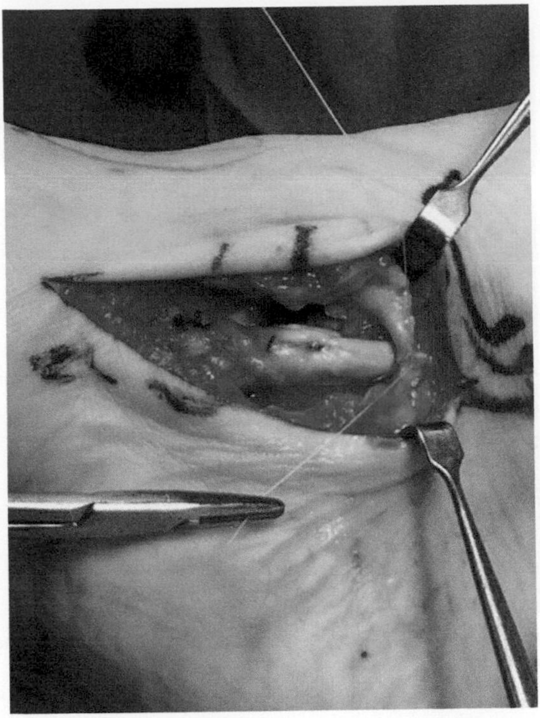

Fig. 9. The tendon was further tubularized, then subcutaneous and skin closure.

Low-lying muscle mass of the peroneus brevis was noted and was excised with cutting cautery. Each of the tendons were débrided. The Artelon implant was sandwiched within the peroneal brevis tendon for reinforcement, and the tendon was retubularized (**Fig. 11**).

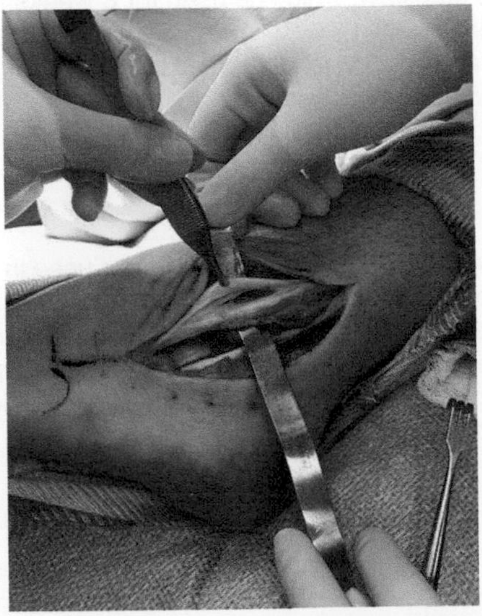

Fig. 10. Dissection revealed a split thickness tear and tenosynovitis of the peroneus brevis tendon and thickening, tenosynovitis and interstitial tear of the peroneus longus tendon.

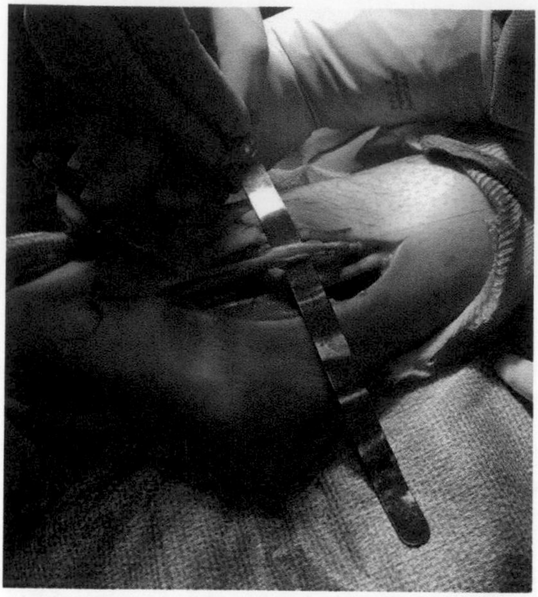

Fig. 11. The Artelon implant was placed internally for reinforcement and the tendon was retubularized. (*Courtesy of* Artelon, Marietta, GA.)

The peroneus longus tendon was retubularized using nonabsorbable suture. Next, a modified Brostrom procedure was performed with the use of an anchor system. The patient was placed in a bivalve below-knee fiberglass cast and was nonweight bearing with the assistance of crutches. At 4 weeks after surgery, he was transitioned into a CAM walker partial weight bearing with crutches, and at 5 weeks after surgery, he discontinued the use of crutches. Seven weeks after surgery the patient was placed in an ankle stabilizer, which he used for 8 weeks and started an 8-week course of physical therapy. By 11 weeks after surgery, the patient returned to full function and was cleared to return to work on his feet without complication. Minimal swelling was noted throughout the postoperative course as well as minimal postoperative pain.

SUMMARY

This article has described 3 cases in which Artelon was used in the repair of the Achilles tendon, posterior tibial tendon, and peroneal tendon injuries. Artelon is a novel and useful alternative for reinforcement of tendon repairs compared with autografts or allografts. These 3 case study patients were all able to return to preinjury activity levels without limitation. At this point, the authors found no complications related to the graft and had good outcomes from all 3 cases.

REFERENCES

1. Heikkinen J, Lantto I, Flinkkila T, et al. Augmented compared with nonaugmented surgical repair after total Achilles tendon rupture. Results of a prospective randomized trial with thirteen or more years of follow-up. J Bone Joint Surg Am 2016;98:85–92.

2. Aktas S, Kocaoglu B, Nalbantoglu U, et al. End-to-end versus augmented repair in the treatment of acute Achilles tendon ruptures. J Foot Ankle Surg 2007;46: 336–40.
3. Ofili K, Pollard J, Schuberth J. The neglected Achilles tendon rupture with repaired allograft: a review of 14 cases. J Foot Ankle Surg 2016;55:1245–8.
4. Jennings A, Sefton G. Chronic rupture of tendo Achilles. Long-term results of operative management using polyester tape. J Bone Joint Surg Br 2002;84(3):361–3.
5. Krause J, Brodskey J. Peroneus brevis tendon tears: pathophysiology, surgical reconstruction, and clinical results. Foot Ankle Int 1998;19(5):271–9.
6. Mook WR, Parekh SG, Nunley JA. Allograft reconstruction of peroneal tendons: operative technique and clinical outcomes. Foot Ankle Int 2013;34(9):1212–20.
7. Rapley JH, Crates J, Barber A. Mid-substance peroneal tendon defects augmented with an acellular dermal matrix allograft. Foot Ankle Int 2010;31: 136–40.
8. Rosenburg ZS. Chronic rupture of posterior tibial tendon. Clin Podiatr Med Surg 1999;16(3):423–38.
9. Vulcano E, Deland JT, Ellis SJ. Approach and treatment of the adult acquired flatfoot deformity. Curr Rev Musculoskelet Med 2013;6(4):294–303.
10. Fleischli JG, Fleischli JW, Laughlin TJ. Treatment of posterior tibial tendon dysfunction with tendon procedures from the posterior muscle group. Clin Podiatr Med Surg 1999;16(3):453–70.
11. Myerson MS, Corrigan J. Treatment of posterior tibial tendon dysfunction with flexor digitorum longus tendon transfer and calcaneal osteotomy. Orthopedics 1996;19(5):383–8.
12. Gazdag AR, Cracchiolo A 3rd. Rupture of the posterior tibial tendon:evaluation of injury of the spring ligament and clinical assessment of tendon transfer and ligament repair. J Bone Joint Surg AM 1997;79(5):675–81.
13. Janis LR, Wagner JT, Kravitz RD, et al. Posterior tibial tendon rupture: classification, modified surgical repair and retrospective study. J Foot Ankle Surg 1993;32: 2–13.
14. Helal BM. Cobb repair for tibialis posterior rupture. J Foot Surg 1990;29(4): 349–52.
15. Weiler A, Peters G, Mäurer J, et al. Biomechanical properties and vascularity of an anterior cruciate ligament graft can be predicted by contrast-enhanced magnetic resonance imaging. A two year study of sheep. Am J Sports Med 2001; 26(6):751–61.
16. Clancy WG Jr, Narechama RG, Rosenberg RD, et al. Anterior and posterior cruciate ligament reconstruction in rhesus monkeys. J Bone Joint Surg Am 1981; 63(8):1270–84.
17. Fu F, Bennett CH, Lattermann C, et al. Current trends in anterior cruciate ligament reconstruction. Part 1: biology and biomechanics of reconstruction. Am J Sports Med 1999;27(6):821–30.
18. Rading J, Peterson L. Clinical experience with the Leeds-Keio artificial ligament in anterior cruciate ligament reconstruction. A prospective two-year follow-up study. Am J Sports Med 1995;23(3):316–9.
19. Wredmark T, Engstrom B. Five-year results of anterior cruciate ligament reconstruction with the Stryker Dacron high-strength ligament. Knee Surg Sports Traumatol Arthrosc 1993;1(2):71–5.
20. Engström B, Wredmark T, Westblad P. Patellar tendon or Leeds-Keio graft in the surgical treatment of anterior cruciate ligament ruptures. Intermediate results. Clin Orthop Relat Res 1993;295:190–7.

21. Denti M, Bigoni M, Dodaro G, et al. Long-term results of the Leeds-Keio anterior cruciate ligament reconstruction. Knee Surg Sports Traumatol Arthrosc 1995; 3(2):75–7.
22. Pattee GA, Friedman M. A review of autogenous intraarticular reconstruction of the anterior cruciate ligament prosthetic ligament reconstruction of the knee. In: Friedman MJ, Ferkel RD, editors. Prosthetic ligament reconstruction of the knee. Philadelphia: Elsevier Saunders; 1988. p. 22–8.
23. Puddu G, Cipolla M, Cerullo G, et al. Anterior cruciate ligament reconstruction and augmentation with PDS graft. Clin Sports Med 1993;12(1):13–24.
24. Gretzer C, Emanuelsson L, Liljensten E, et al. The inflammatory cell influx and cytokines changes during transition from acute inflammation to fibrous repair around implanted materials. J Biomater Sci Polym Ed 2006;17(6):669–87.
25. Giza E, Frizzell L, Farac R, et al. Augmented tendon Achilles repair using a tissue reinforcement scaffold: a biomechanical study. Foot Ankle Int 2011;32(5):S545–9.
26. Gisselfalt K, Edberg B, Flodin P. Synthesis and properties of degradable poly(urethane urea)s to be used for ligament reconstructions. Biomacromolecules 2002;3:951–8.
27. Liljensten E, Gisselfält K, Edberg B, et al. Studies of polyurethane urea bands for ACL reconstruction. J Mater Sci Mater Med 2002;13:351–9.

Near-Infrared Spectroscopy Imaging for Assessing Skin and Wound Oxygen Perfusion

Adam S. Landsman, DPM, PhD[a,*], Darrell Barnhart, BS[b],
Michael Sowa, PhD[b]

KEYWORDS

- Near-infrared spectroscopy • NIRS • Wound perfusion • Healing rate
- Oxygenated hemoglobin • Tissue oxygenation • Tissue oxygen perfusion

KEY POINTS

- One of the most important aspects in assessment of wound closure and skin viability is blood supply.
- Measurement of blood supply has continually evolved over the last 30 years, from simply palpating pulses to angiography to peripheral circulatory measurements based on skin perfusion.
- Light-based systems have provided a new way to evaluate the delicate peripheral oxygenation of superficial tissues.

INTRODUCTION

Without a doubt, among the most important aspects in assessment of wound closure and skin viability is blood supply. Blood carries nutrients to the site and removes waste. It plays a role in every aspect of tissue life. Measurement of blood supply has continually evolved over the last 30 years, from simply palpating pulses to angiography to peripheral circulatory measurements based on skin perfusion. The evaluation of skin perfusion becomes much more complex due to the tiny and diffuse nature of the capillary beds.

The Ankle-Brachial Index and angiography give little useful information when it comes to evaluating blood flow to the skin. Historically, patients may have good macroscopic blood flow and yet still may have poor skin perfusion, which can be

Disclosures: A. Landsman serves as the Chief Medical Officer for Kent Imaging. M. Sowa and D. Barnhart are employed by Kent Imaging.

[a] Division of Podiatric Surgery, Department of Surgery, Cambridge Health Alliance, Harvard Medical School, 1493 Cambridge Street, Floor 2, Cambridge, MA 02139, USA; [b] Kent Imaging, 804B 16 Avenue, SW, Calgary, AB T2R 0S9, Canada
* Corresponding author.
E-mail address: alandsman@cha.harvard.edu

Clin Podiatr Med Surg 35 (2018) 343–355
https://doi.org/10.1016/j.cpm.2018.02.005

attributed to basement membrane thickening in patients with diabetes and to issues such as microembolism in patients with a history of atherosclerotic disease.

Light-based systems have provided a new way to evaluate the delicate peripheral oxygenation of superficial tissues. Pulse oximetry (S_pO2) systems are routinely found in operating rooms and are a staple for monitoring oxygenation levels during anesthesia. This simple diode-receptor combination attaches to a finger and measures changes in oxygenation levels in the larger arteries. Similarly, plastic surgeons have relied on local probes that can be attached directly to a skin flap to monitor flow to 1 point within the flap. Flow is calculated using an algorithm and is expressed in tissue perfusion units, which does not actually relate to a volumetric measure but rather a relative assessment of perfusion. Both modalities have 2 significant limitations. The first is that they require direct contact with the tissues. This may be problematic in cases in which there is concern about an infection. The second issue is that they provide information from only a single point, without providing any information about adjacent areas.

To measure greater areas of tissue, an intravenous dye, indocyanine green (ICG) can be administered. It has a peak spectral absorption of around 800 nm, and can be viewed when a specialized light source and camera are used to view the tissues shortly after administration. Typically, this process is done within the operating room suite, allowing real-time viewing of the tissues as they are being perfused. Although this system is highly capable of providing a detailed image of the superficial tissue circulation, it has significant limitations. The test must be conducted in an operating room suite, adding significant costs. The test cannot be immediately repeated, which is problematic if taking an image, adjusting some aspect influencing perfusion, and then repeating the image to determine if the adjustment had any effect. For example, if a patient had reflex sympathetic dystrophy with autonomically controlled vasoconstriction, the image would show reduced perfusion. Then, if a nerve block is performed, one would expect to see resultant vasodilation but this would not be possible with an ICG system. A second limitation is the physical size of the device. A typical ICG-based system is on a large cart that requires a significant amount of space and coordination to operate.

Thermography is another alternative that may give some indication about the level of peripheral circulation. Historically, warm tissues are well-perfused, whereas colder tissues are not. Although thermography can be used to assess peripheral circulation indirectly, the images typically lack detail, and are highly susceptible to changes in room temperature and the patient's level of comfort. Consequently, thermographic images are highly irreproducible.

More recently, near-infrared spectroscopy (NIRS) has become available. This technique is based on the transmission of near-infrared light onto the skin surface. Some portions of the light are absorbed, whereas other portions are reflected. The device used in this study is an imaging NIRS device (Kent KD203, Kent Imaging, Calgary, AB, Canada), emitting a series of illuminating flashes of near-infrared light between 600 and 1000 nm. Light around 750 nm is predominantly absorbed by unbound hemoglobin, whereas light around 850 nm is predominantly absorbed by hemoglobin bound to oxygen. By measuring the relative absorption of near-infrared light around those key wavelengths, the ratio of oxygenated to oxygenation plus deoxygenated hemoglobin can be determined. Well-perfused tissues will have a higher percent of oxygenated hemoglobin than poorly perfused skin (**Fig. 1**).

Spectroscopy systems that use near-infrared light to determine hemoglobin oxygenation have the benefit of sampling tissue more deeply compared with their visible light counterparts. This is particularly the case in the presence of higher

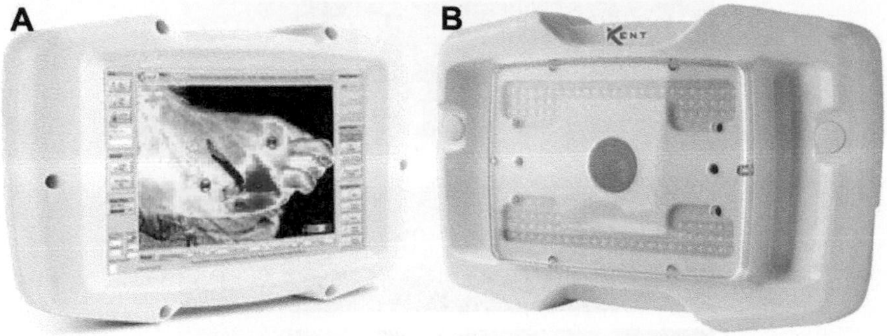

Fig. 1. Kent Imaging NIRS device (*A*). Front of Kent camera showing light-emitting diodes and camera lens (*B*). (*Courtesy of* Kent Imaging Calgary, Alberta, Canada).

epidermal melanin content. Visible light is highly attenuated by melanin, whereas near-infrared light is less affected. Thus, visible light devices are challenged to sample beyond the epidermal melanin layer in darker skin.

To establish the accuracy of this measurement technique, Bowen and colleagues[1] looked at the correlation between measurements taken using NIRS and trans cutaneous oxygen perfusion (TCPO2) in patients with chronic wounds. They took simultaneous measurements on 20 subjects, and found a correlation coefficient of 0.92 and r^2 equals 0.84, indicating that the NIRS correlated well with TCPO2. They also noted that there were some significant advantages to using NIRS, including lower cost and its noncontact nature, compared with the need for a TCPO2 probe, which must actually touch the skin being assessed. The investigators also noted the faster sampling time with NIRS, approximately 2 minutes versus 90 minutes with TCPO2.

Using an array of infrared emitters, the NIRS device can capture data from large areas of skin. The device used in this study is able to capture oxygen perfusion data over an area of approximately 150 cm^2. Over the 8 seconds it takes to collect and display data, it captures a JPEG clinical image, as well as the images showing oxygenated and deoxygenated hemoglobin. Using an algorithm to calculate the ratios, the images can be overlaid to determine the oxygen perfusion of any area within the field of view. Simply touching a portion of the screen instantaneously displays the ratio of oxygenated to oxygenated plus deoxygenated hemoglobin within an area of approximately 0.2 cm^2 (**Fig. 2**).

In this study, NIRS was used to evaluate skin oxygen perfusion. These data were used to draw some conclusions about the correlation between the level of tissue oxygenation and the ability to heal a wound. Other clinical applications were also explored, including an assessment of skin flaps and the predictive value of NIRS for flap survival.

EVALUATION OF DIABETIC FOOT ULCERS

Foot ulcers are among the most common complications among patients with diabetes, particularly in the presence of neuropathy and/or peripheral vascular disease. Regardless of the specific etiologic factor causing the ulcer to form, vascular perfusion is essential for healing. In this evaluation, a group of subjects with diabetes and wounds were followed to determine if NIRS had any predictive value for determining the probability of closure. This study builds on the work by Livingston,[2] which was presented as an abstract but never published due to the death of the investigator shortly

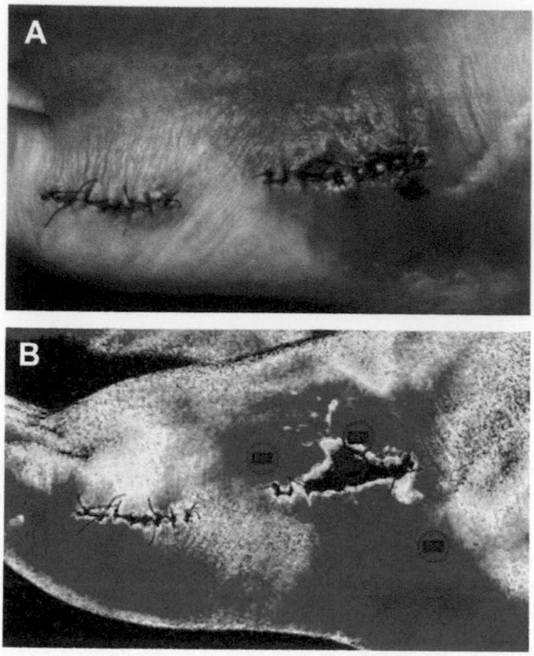

Fig. 2. Skin slough following excision of lipoma. Immediate clinical picture shows a well-coapted wound, with some evidence of bruising (*A*). However, the NIRS image shows the ischemia above the incision line (11%) (*B*). This area did go on to a full-thickness slough.

after the preliminary work was completed. In his preliminary study, Livingston found that when the ratio of oxygenated to oxygenated plus deoxygenated hemoglobin was lower than 40%, the risk of wounds not healing increased dramatically. Therefore, in the current study, the authors paid particular attention to cases in which the ratio was less than or equal to 40%. In addition, we have observed that the percentage of oxygenated hemoglobin can be limited to the area within the wound margin or can spread to the areas surrounding the wound. Therefore, the impact of perfusion in the adjacent areas was also examined.

Finally, the accuracy of the displayed values partially depend on the interference of pigmentation when trying to penetrate through the skin. Pigmentation is usually described according to the Fitzpatrick scale,[3] ranging from Fitzpatrick 1 (very light coloration) to Fitzpatrick 6, which is the darkest (**Table 1**). All light-based systems must take pigmentation into account when determining absorption and reflection, and will use an algorithm for compensating for melanin levels.

The following case series illustrate some of the critical issues associated with NIRS. In particular, the ability to predict wound healing and flap survival are the primary focus of this research.

Case #1: Predicting Surgical Wound Dehiscence

A 38-year-old woman had a 3 cm soft tissue mass excised from the dorsal lateral aspect of her left foot. The lesion appeared to be a ganglion and was located superficial to the deep fascia. **Fig. 2** shows the patient immediately after surgery, with sutures in place. Clinically, there is some slight bruising apparent but no evidence of

Table 1
Options for treatment of ischemic changes

Issue	Treatment
• Ischemia along incision line	• Reposition sutures • Loosen tension
• Ischemia extending away from incision	• Hyperbaric oxygenation
• Poor perfusion of wound bed	• Surgical debridement • Negative-pressure therapy • Warm room environment
• Venous congestion	• Nitroglycerin paste
• Ischemic areas surrounding the wound	• Vascular intervention to restore or improve overall blood flow

ischemia (**Fig. 2**A). However, the NIRS image showed 11% oxygen saturation to the central portion of the incision (**Fig. 2**B). The adjacent tissues show excellent tissue oxygen saturation (S_tO_2) with values ranging from 69% to 84% S_tO_2. The patient is a Fitzpatrick 2 to 3, so no melanin correction was required. Seven days after this image was captured, the surgical wound dehisced and there was a full-thickness slough along the incision line.

Due to the size of the wound and the exposure of the deep fascia, a split-thickness skin graft was required to achieve closure. Examination of the skin graft shortly after application revealed a secured graft with minimal perfusion noted. Over time, the graft slowly incorporated, and the improvement in wound bed perfusion was apparent with the NIRS.

Case #2: Determining the Level and Timing of Amputation

A 70-year-old man with diabetes presented with gangrenous changes to his hallux. NIRS images suggested a clear line of demarcation in the area just proximal to the metatarsal phalangeal joint. Several images were captured over a period of 3 weeks, with no notable changes in the line of demarcation and with relatively poor levels of oxygenation at the margin itself (**Fig. 3**A). Based on the stability of the demarcation line, the decision was made to perform an amputation of the gangrenous hallux, as well as resection of the first metatarsal head.

Immediately following the surgery, the clinical picture of the foot seemed to show an excellent outcome, with good coloration of the skin along the wound margin. However, the NIRS image clearly showed a different story (**Fig. 3**B). In this image, one could appreciate the drop in percentage of S_tO_2 to only 18%. Not surprisingly, the wound dehisced approximately 1 week later. The foot began to show signs of ischemia, with widening of the area of low S_tO_2. Ultimately, gangrenous changes started to appear, extending proximally and laterally. At this point, the decision was made to proceed on to a transmetatarsal amputation.

Three weeks after the initial procedure, the transmetatarsal amputation was performed without complication. Clinical examination of the foot appeared to show good coloration, and the wound remained well-coapted. NIRS taken at the same time showed some slight decrease in perfusion along the incision line, with some areas going as low as 43% and 48% S_tO_2 (**Fig. 3**C). Considering 40% as the benchmark for adequate oxygenation for healing, it was not surprising that this wound did go on to heal completely without complication.

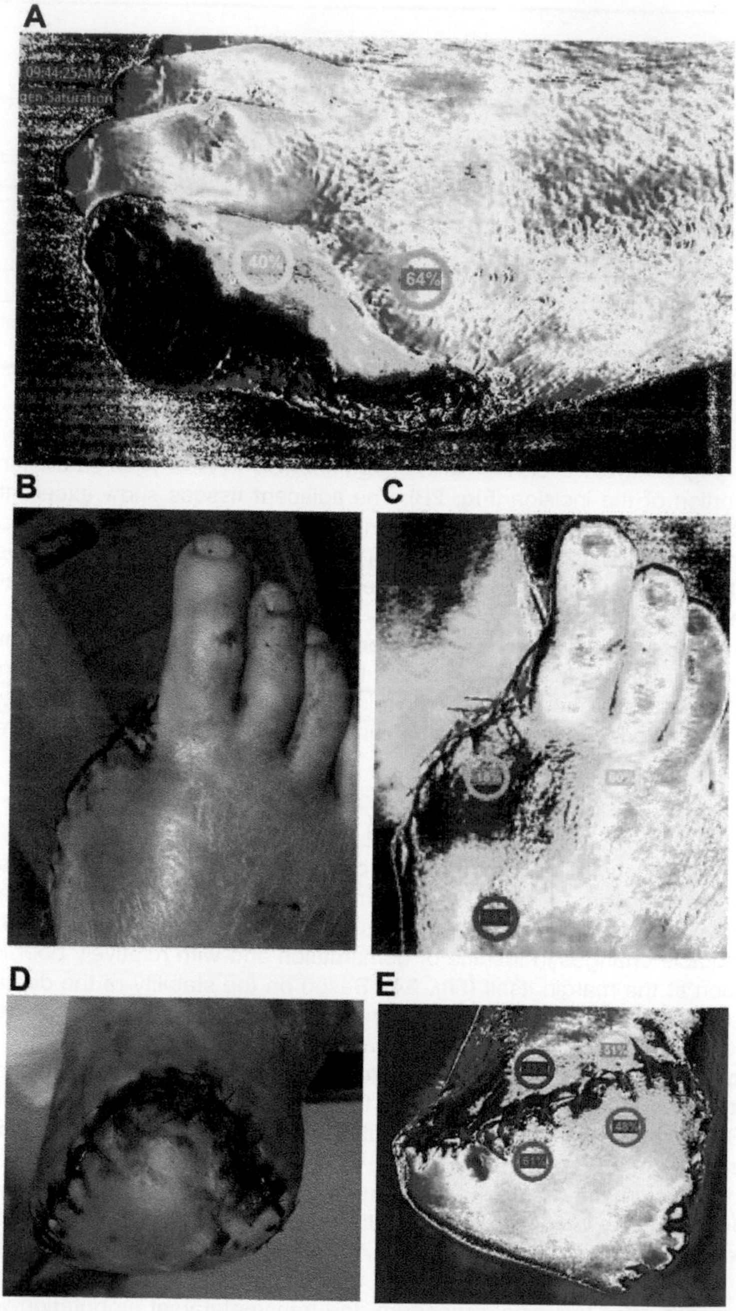

Fig. 3. Evaluation of skin demarcation following gangrene and amputation. This patient had gangrenous changes to the hallux and, based on NIRS images, the decision was made to resect to the level of the first metatarsal phalangeal joint (*A*). Initially, the clinical appearance of the foot was good (*B*) but the NIRS image tells another story with ischemic changes (18%) along the incision line that ultimately led to total dehiscence of the closure (*C*). Due to the extent of the damage, ultimately, a transmetatarsal amputation was needed (*D*), which resulted in much better perfusion along the incision line, and this did go on to full healing (*E*).

Case #3: Skin Graft Incorporation

A 67-year-old woman presented with a chronic ankle ulceration that was present for nearly 2 years. She had treatments with multiple biologic and living cell products with progressive worsening of the wound. Ultimately, her wound deteriorated to reach the level of the medial malleolus and exposed periosteum. After her initial presentation, an NIRS image showed very low levels of oxygenation, consistent with this relatively dysvascular tissue. She was taken to the operating room where debridement was performed, to the level of bone, and an array of small holes was drilled into the bone with a Kirschner wire to stimulate bleeding. Following copious irrigation, a cryopreserved split-thickness skin allograft was applied (TheraSkin, Soluble Systems, Newport News, VA, USA).

One week after application, the patient returned to the clinic. Examination of the wound was inconclusive concerning whether or not the graft had become incorporated (**Fig.** 4A). However, an NIRS image clearly demonstrated not only excellent perfusion of the wound bed but also integration of the graft (**Fig.** 4B). Four weeks later, the graft was fully incorporated into the wound bed and a second graft was applied. The wound went on to full closure 8 weeks after initial debridement and graft application.

Case#4: Gangrenous Changes in a Toe

A very common scenario is the presentation of a toe with wet gangrene. In most cases, amputation is eminent to reduce the risk of prolonged drainage and exacerbation of infection. Images taken (**Fig.** 5A, C) show the clinical picture, with obvious destruction to the tip of the toe. However, the question was how far the damage extended.

In the NIRS images (**Fig.** 5B, D), it is apparent that the damage does not extend beyond the proximal interphalangeal joint. A partial amputation of the toe was performed and the wound went on to heal without complications.

Case #5: Deep Laceration of Skin to the Toe

This patient presented to the emergency department with a deep laceration to the dorsum of the hallux and second toe. Initially, the elevated skin appeared to be dusky and it was questionable whether or not the skin flap would survive. Following a cleansing of the area, the flap was reapproximated to the wound bed using

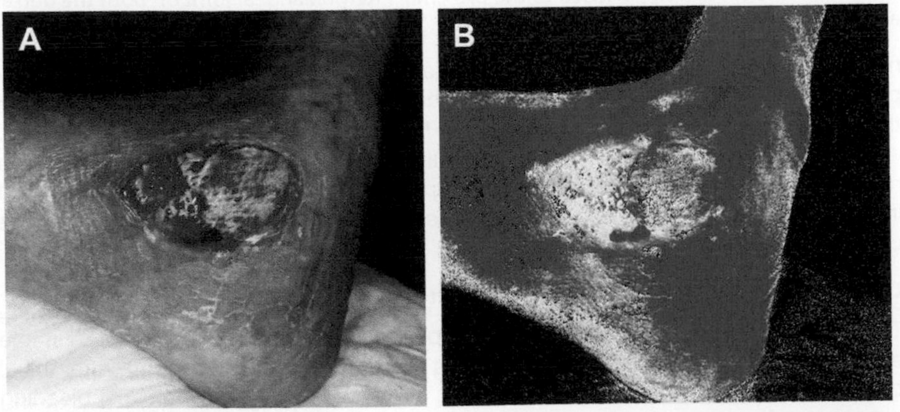

Fig. 4. Full-thickness venous ulceration to the medial malleolus. The skin graft is showing minimal evidence of integration on the clinical picture (*A*). However, the NIRS image clearly demonstrates excellent perfusion of the skin graft, which did go on to complete closure (*B*).

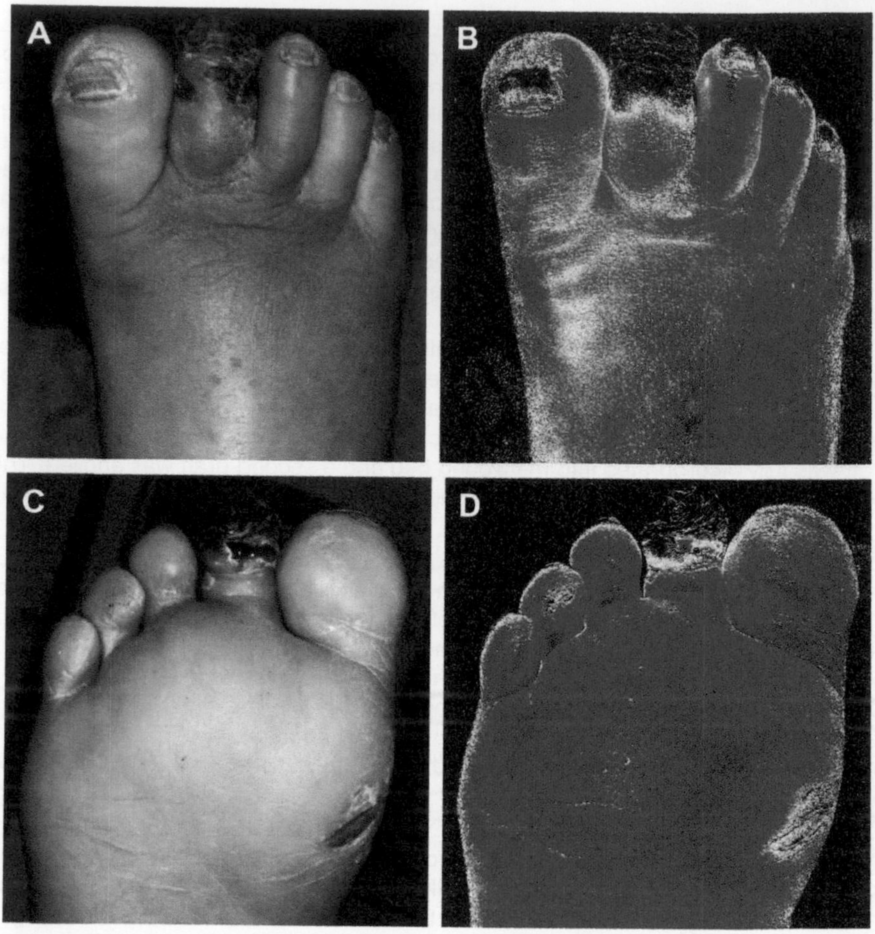

Fig. 5. Determining level of perfusion in the presence of a gangrenous toe. Clinically, the level of demarcation of the second digit is poorly defined (*A, C*) but the NIRS image clearly shows that the toe is well-perfused to the proximal interphalangeal joint on both the dorsal and plantar surfaces (*B, D*).

monofilament suture. NIRS demonstrated a large area where the flap was poorly perfused over the hallux. The patient was instructed to reduce activity level, keep the foot elevated, avoid ice to the area, and leave the bandages in place (**Fig. 6**A, B).

Subsequently, the patient returned to clinic 1 week later and the imaging was repeated. It was apparent that the skin flap was surviving, and that perfusion had improved (**Fig. 6**C, D). The final outcome 3 weeks after the original injury was complete closure of the wound (**Fig. 6**E, F).

Case #6: Plantar Skin Graft with Subsequent Revascularization

The patient presented with sloughing of the plantar mid-arch area of the foot. A stable eschar was present but wound healing was not progressing. One month after initial presentation, the eschar was debrided and, at the time of surgery, minimal bleeding was noted from the plantar surface. A split-thickness skin allograft was applied and NIRS images demonstrated poor oxygenation of the surrounding tissues (**Fig. 7**A, B). Two weeks after angioplasty imaging showed restored flow to the foot.

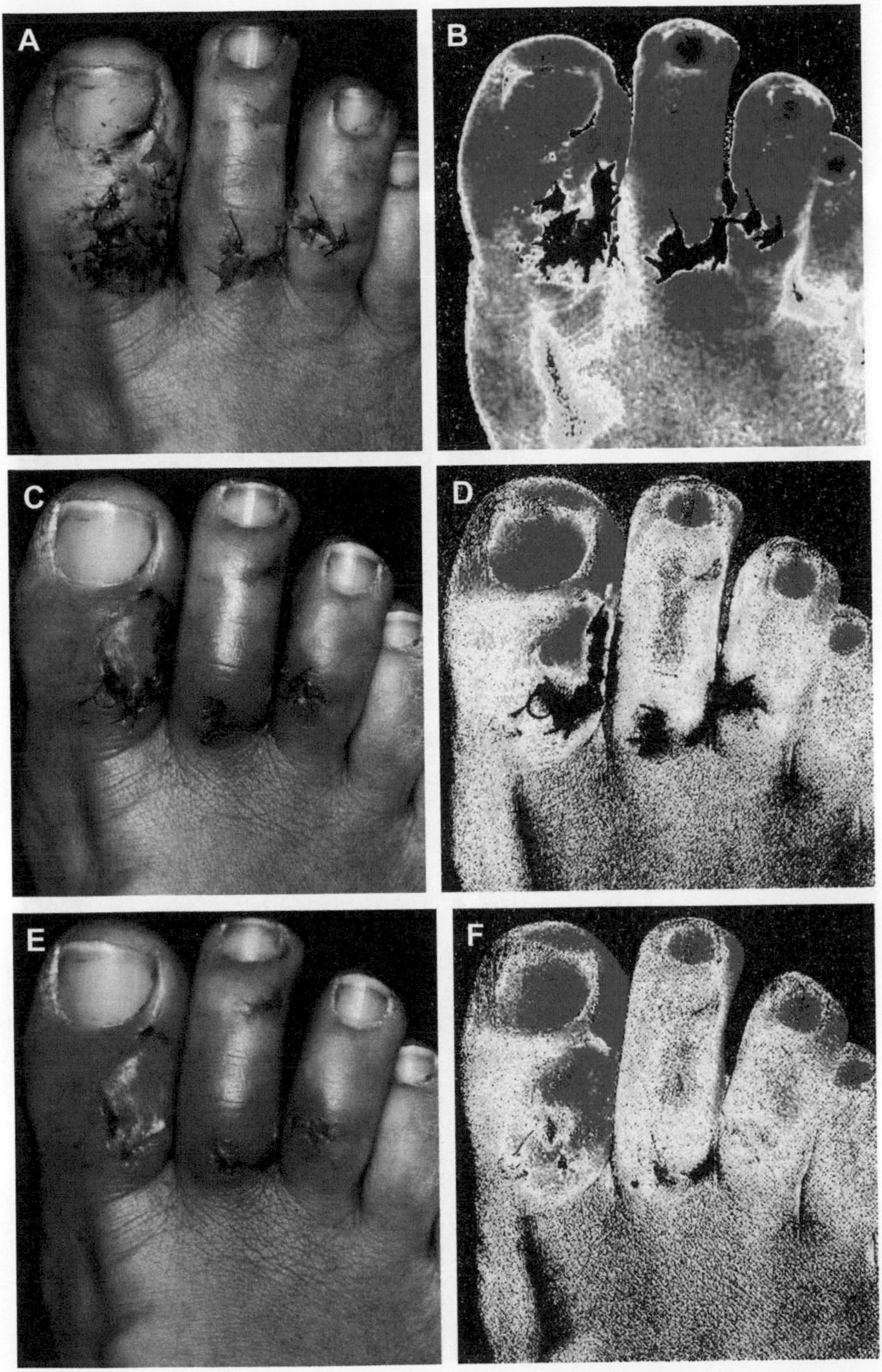

Fig. 6. Laceration of skin. The initial laceration (*A*) along with the NIRS image (*B*) show poor perfusion of the laceration but excellent perfusion in the adjacent tissue. One week later, the skin is adhering well (*C*) and the increase in perfusion is evident in the flap (*D*). Two weeks later, sutures are removed, and the skin appears to have survived (*E*). The NIRS image also demonstrates excellent oxygenation of the tissues (*F*).

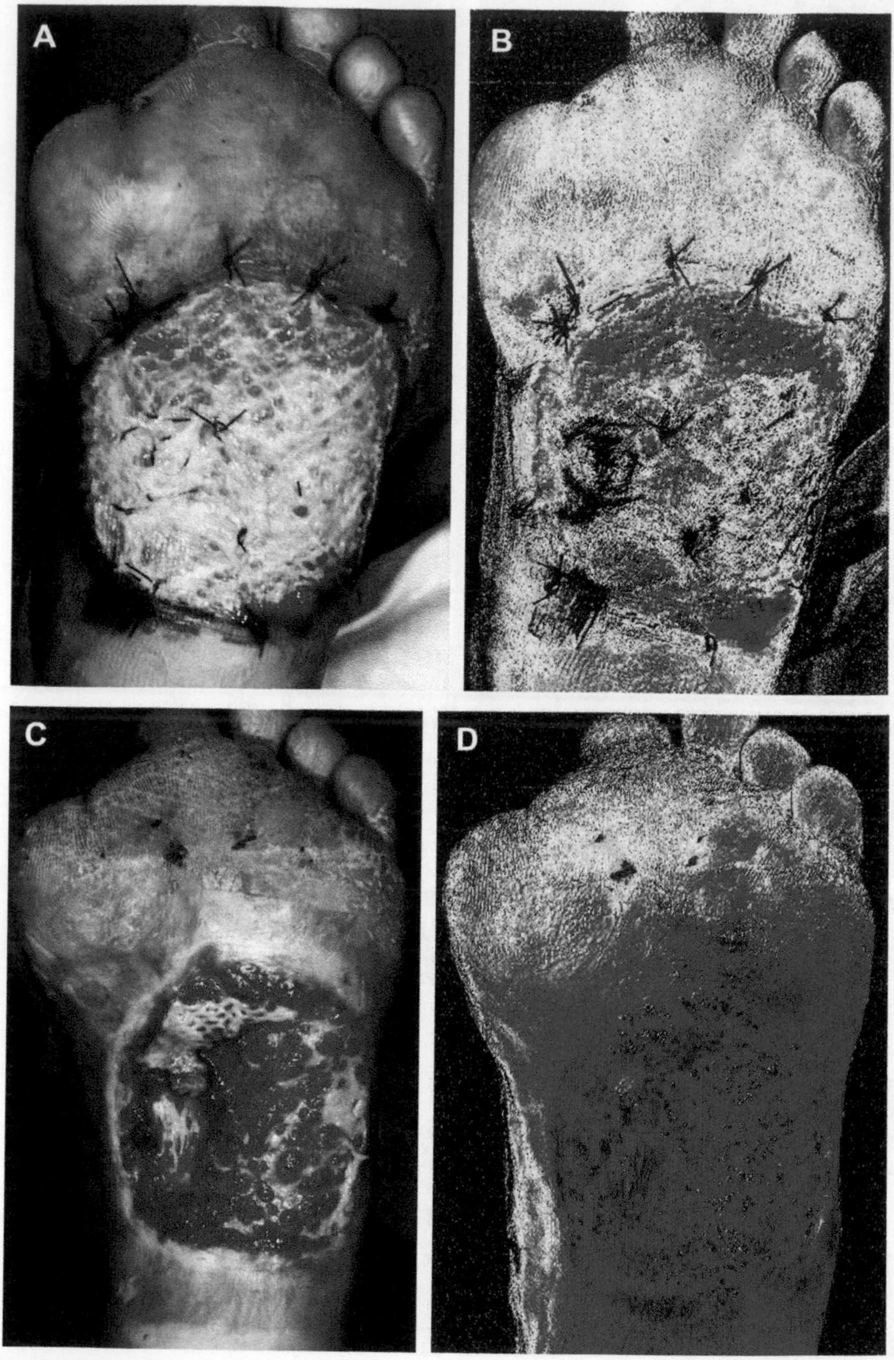

Fig. 7. Vascular intervention to save a skin flap. Clinical image (*A*) and NIRS image (*B*) demonstrate several areas of graft integration but there was concern on the NIRS image for ischemia over adjacent areas on the plantar surface. Two weeks after angioplasty, the clinical image shows increase in granulation tissue throughout the graft (*C*) and the NIRS image illustrates the improved perfusion of the entire plantar surface of the foot (*D*).

One can appreciate the change in perfusion to the plantar skin (**Fig. 7**D), as well as the improvement in granulation tissue and graft incorporation that accompanied the improvement in flow (**Fig. 7**C).

DISCUSSION

NIRS is an invaluable tool for evaluation of tissue oxygenation and perfusion. In the authors' series, there were several trends observed. The previous study by Bowen and colleagues[1] clearly demonstrated that the oxygenation levels determined from NIRS correlated precisely with TCPO2 measurements, with the added advantages of more rapid assessment, without the need for patient contact, in addition to the ability to assess the condition of the skin over a much larger area.

Like all light-based systems, NIRS relies on the ability to differentiate between the color of oxygenated and deoxygenated hemoglobin in the face of various levels of melanin in the skin. The ability to gather accurate data in more darkly pigmented individuals becomes more elusive and depends on the algorithms used to filter the data, as well as the wavelengths of light chosen. Near-infrared light, like that used with the Kent Imaging device, is able to penetrate more deeply into the tissues than visible light systems, giving a much more accurate determination of the oxygenation levels of the wound bed and surrounding skin.

One limitation to the NIRS device is the need for measuring reflected light. Nearly all body parts have some slight curvature to their surface. When the curvature becomes extreme, such as along the edge of a foot, the images appear to show lower levels of oxygenation. This is an obvious artifact of making measurements over larger areas. A strong advantage to using a fast handheld device, such as that used in this study, is that it becomes very easy to take several images from different points of view to more accurately assess the percentages of oxygenation while eliminating the edge effects. This device is very light in weight, and can easily be held in a position that is parallel to the surface of interest, and can be used to take pictures from the top, bottom, and sides. This becomes much more difficult when trying to image curved surfaces with a stand-mounted device.

In the clinical setting, measurement of tissue oxygenation is useful for giving insights to the potential for healing based not only on the levels of oxygenation within the wound bed but also in the surrounding areas. In the authors' clinical experience, we have found NIRS to be highly useful for predicting flap failure and surgical wound dehiscence. Immediate testing of tissues following surgery in which the tissues appeared to be healthy and viable clinically, often gave accurate clues of potential future problems when the NIRS images were examined. In fact, we found that reduced levels of tissue oxygenation may predict as far as 7 days in advance when a flap is likely to fail. By knowing this far in advance that there is a potential problem with a surgical wound or skin flap, several steps can be taken to protect the tissues (see **Table 1**).

Previously, it was reported that a tissue oxygenation percentage greater than 40% is required to achieve wound healing, depending also on the levels of oxygenation of the adjacent surrounding tissues. The authors' experiences concur that oxygenation levels of around 40% are significant. Although we have seen wounds that have closed with oxygenation levels into the 30% range, this usually will occur only if the surrounding tissues are well-perfused and the wound is relatively small. Conversely, we have seen wounds with oxygenation levels in the 50% and even 60% levels that were nonprogressive but these wounds were usually larger and deeper. In cases in which there is an overall decreased level of oxygenation, surgical intervention to restore blood flow may be indicated. Conversely, if the immediate area of the wound appears to be well-perfused, further intervention may not be necessary.

SUMMARY

New biologic wound treatments are changing the way that clinicians think about achieving healing. The addition of collagen, growth factors, hyaluronic acid, and living cell therapy have given the clinician new tools for addressing deficits in the healing process. Similarly, diagnostic tools to assess wound bed pathologic conditions are also evolving and now include measures for matrix metalloproteases (MMPs), pH, and quick tests for biofilms. Pressure and temperature transducers built into shoes, or even floor mats, can add further information to predict who may develop or fail to heal a wound.

Of all of the factors that influence wound healing, oxygenated blood flow is probably the most critical. Without blood flow, there is no mechanism for delivering nutrients and removing waste products. Furthermore, there is no nourishment of these tissues, which are often compromised by infection, and other issues. With time, the ability to interpret the effect of perfusion, both macroscopically and microscopically, continues to improve. From simple methods that use measurement of pulses and handheld Doppler, to more sophisticated techniques, such as fluorescent and radiopaque dye injection, the ability to assess vascular insufficiency and treat these problems continues to evolve.

NIS is a natural extension in the evolution of perfusion measurement. The current device illustrates the high quality of the data that can be collected, showing details in perfusion that can be determined across the entire surface of skin in increments of only a millimeter or 2. In the future, clinicians and scientists will become better at understanding the direct correlation between local oxygenation levels and determining the effect on wound healing.

Future applications for NIRS will certainly include early detection of MMPs that can stimulate angiogenesis but also cause periwound inflammation when present at excessive levels. Similarly, wounds that are infected may show increased periwound perfusion. Ischemia in the tissues can easily be detected before it is clinically apparent and will help determine the presence of microvascular disease, as well as serve as a signal to identify patients in need of vascular intervention. Imaging of the wound surface will also help assess when adequate debridement has been achieved.

Although the current study focused on the use of NIRS for applications related to wound healing, the value of NIRS is much greater. General surgeons who are performing anastomosis following bowel resection, for example, can image the surgical site intraoperatively to assess the quality of their repair. Similarly, plastic surgeons can use NIRS as a tool for assessing tissue perfusion in areas where sloughing is common, such as with various types of skin flaps. Physicians who administer oxygen in hyperbaric chambers may even be able to assess both the value of the current treatment, as well as the longer persisting benefits of this modality. Ultimately, NIRS will be seen is a way to detect the transition between normal, well-perfused tissues and abnormal tissues. The ramifications for this extend far beyond the assessment of wounds.

REFERENCES

1. Bowen RE, Treadwell GRN, Goodwin MRRT. Correlation of near infrared spectroscopy measurements of tissue oxygen saturation with transcutaneous pO2 in patients with chronic wounds. SM Vasc Med 2016;1(2):2016.

2. Livingston M. Multispectral oximetry imaging readings with associated healing trajectory. Document on file with Kent Imaging. 2015. Available at: http://www.kentimaging.com/research/.
3. Sachdeva S. Fitzpatrick skin typing: applications in dermatology. Indian J Dermatol Venereol Leprol 2009;75(1):93–6.

Special Article

Randomized, Prospective, Blinded-Enrollment, Head-To-Head Venous Leg Ulcer Healing Trial Comparing Living, Bioengineered Skin Graft Substitute (Apligraf) with Living, Cryopreserved, Human Skin Allograft (TheraSkin)

Michael A. Towler, MD[a,*], Elaine W. Rush, RN, BS, CWOCN[a], Melissa K. Richardson, MD[a], Calvin L. Williams, PhD[b]

KEYWORDS

- Venous leg ulcer • VLU • Venous stasis ulcer • TheraSkin • Apligraf • Biologic graft • Chronic wound healing

KEY POINTS

- There was a statistically significant 42.2% decrease in cost for the appropriate graft sizes in the TheraSkin cohort ($2495.33/subject) compared with the Apligraf cohort ($4316.67/subject), even though the initial wound sizes were not significantly different between groups.
- Although there were higher venous leg ulcer (VLU) healing rates with the TheraSkin cohort compared with the Apligraf cohort at both12 weeks (93.3% vs 75.0%) and 20 weeks (93.3% vs 83.3%), these healing rate differences were not statistically significant.

Continued

Disclosure Statement: The authors have no conflicts of interest. They have no financial relationship with Soluble Systems, LLC, LifeNet Health, Inc, or Organogenesis, Inc. This research was performed without author funding. In addition, neither the Bon Secours St Francis Wound Healing Center (where the research was conducted) or its affiliated Bon Secours St Francis Hospital were compensated in any way for this research. Soluble Systems, LLC, Newport News, Virginia, provided administrative assistance to M.A. Towler in obtaining institutional review board (IRB) approval through Western IRB (WIRB) and paid WIRB (Puyallup, WA; Study #1138086; WIRB Pro # 20130425) directly for costs associated with initial IRB approval and annual maintenance.

[a] Bon Secours St Francis Wound Healing Center, Suite 100, 131 Commonwealth Drive, Greenville, SC 29615, USA; [b] Department of Mathematical Sciences, Center for Excellence in Mathematics and Science Education, Clemson University, 0-323 Martin Hall, Clemson, SC 29634-0975, USA

* Corresponding author.

E-mail address: mtowler@charter.net

Clin Podiatr Med Surg 35 (2018) 357–365
https://doi.org/10.1016/j.cpm.2018.02.006

podiatric.theclinics.com

Continued

- There was no statistically significant difference in the number of grafts required to achieve wound closure within limitations of the small sample size presented.
- The use of 1 of these biologics in conjunction with compression therapy is a safe and effective way to treat VLUs.

INTRODUCTION

Chronic venous leg ulcers (VLUs) are responsible for significant morbidity and health care costs worldwide. It is estimated that approximately 1% of populations of developed nations are affected by chronic VLUs.[1] The annual cost of medical intervention for a VLU is reported to be approximately $9600 per wound.[2] The annual payer burden in the United States related to VLUs is estimated to be $14.9 billion.[3]

Biologically active skin graft substitutes, combined with standard compression therapy, have been shown to accelerate wound healing.[4–7] US Food and Drug Administration (FDA)-approved living skin graft substitutes continue to be used as an aid in the healing of refractory VLUs.

This pilot study was undertaken to estimate the relative difference in the effectiveness of 2 widely used living biologic graft options for the treatment of VLUs in a randomized, prospective, head-to-head clinical trial at a single site (Bon Secours St Francis Wound Healing Center, Greenville, SC, USA). They both incorporate viable human skin cells and are both skin graft replacement products. The authors anticipate that data from this pilot study can be useful as a basis for a power calculation to estimate the study size needed for an equivalence or superiority study in the future.

Apligraf (Organogenesis, Canton, MA, USA) is a living, human, bioengineered skin substitute. It was cleared by the FDA as a medical device in 1998 for the treatment of VLUs, and has been widely used with more than 425,000 units of Apligraf supplied to wound care and outpatient centers throughout the United States. Apligraf is supplied as a living, bilayered skin substitute consisting of an outer layer of keratinocytes derived from neonatal foreskin (penile circumcisions) and laminated over a deeper layer of type I bovine collagen impregnated with cultured, foreskin-derived neonatal fibroblasts. According to the Organogenesis Web site (www.apligraf.com), unlike human skin, Apligraf does not contain melanocytes, Langerhans cells, macrophages, lymphocytes, blood vessels, hair follicles, or sweat glands. It is supplied as a circular disc approximately 75 mm in diameter and 0.75 mm thick. It is the only living, bilayered, cell-based product cleared by the FDA for the treatment of both diabetic foot ulcers and VLUs. Apligraf costs approximately $1295 per unit, and each unit has a surface area of 44 cm^2. In a previous study, Apligraf was shown to have a 63% healing rate in VLUs with an average size of 1.33 ($\pm$ 2.69) cm^2 after 26 weeks compared with 49% in a control group.[4]

TheraSkin (procured and processed by LifeNet Health, Virginia Beach, VA, USA, and distributed by Soluble Systems, Inc, Newport News, VA, USA) is a cryopreserved human split-thickness skin allograft harvested within 24 hours postmortem from an organ donor who clears standard safety screenings for organ procurement. When harvested, TheraSkin is washed with antibiotics in accordance with FDA specifications and cryopreserved up to 5 years, until it is delivered on dry ice. It is thawed to room temperature just before application. A previous study has verified the survival of the living cells found in this graft throughout the harvest, cryopreservation, and warming process.[8]

TheraSkin is regulated by the FDA as a human cell, tissue, and cellular and tissue-based product (HCT/P) under section 361 of the Public Health Service Act. It can be used on external acute and chronic wounds, including but not limited to diabetic foot ulcers, VLUs, pressure ulcers, burns, radiation injury, and necrotizing fasciitis, as well as over exposed muscle, tendon, bone, and joint capsule.[5] TheraSkin is available as a 39 cm^2 graft ($1195), a 12 cm^2 graft ($1095), and a 6 cm^2 graft (not used in this study). During the study, we used only the 39 cm^2 and 13 cm^2 graft sizes as determined by the size of the wound being grafted. Each graft is previously fenestrated and can stretch to cover slightly larger areas if needed.

In a retrospective study of 134 VLU subjects with an average wound size of 11.8 ($\pm$ 22.5) cm^2, TheraSkin graft applications to refractory VLUs resulted in healing rates of 60.8% after 12 weeks and 74.6% after 20 weeks.[5]

This pilot study is the first randomized, prospective study comparing these 2 skin substitute graft options in the treatment of VLUs. The study was designed to compare the performance of each skin substitute to assess for differences in healing rates, adverse outcomes, and treatment costs. The data will be used to estimate the relative difference in wound closure and costs, to properly power a larger noninferiority study in the future. It was hypothesized that there was no difference in the healing rates, adverse events, and treatment costs when using TheraSkin with compression therapy compared with an identical treatment protocol that substituted Apligraf for TheraSkin.

To minimize the risk of investigator bias, no honorarium, or other form of payment was received by the investigators. All products were purchased direct from the manufacturers, without any discounts. No payments or other forms of compensation were paid to the subjects. Soluble Systems, LLC, paid the fees associated with the institutional review board (IRB) evaluation directly to Western IRB (WIRB) (study number 1138086; WIRB Pro Number: 20130425).

METHODS

This study was designed as a prospective randomized pilot study in which subjects successfully enrolled in the study were randomized to 1 of 2 cohorts between June 2013 and June 2016. All subjects were required to meet the inclusion and exclusion criteria found in **Table 1**.

Eligible subjects were placed into 1 of the 2 cohorts based on instructions in a randomization envelope. Envelopes were randomized in blocks of 6 and numbered by a research assistant so that they could only be opened in sequence. The investigators were unaware of the block size and were required to open the envelopes in sequence to avoid investigator bias toward either treatment option.

To qualify for participation in this study, a study subject must have had a wound present for at least 30 days that was not responsive to standard of care treatment (compression and local wound care). Subjects could have more than 30 days of conservative treatment before enrollment but 30 days was considered the minimum. This also served as the run-in period, and, therefore, required no prior treatment with biologics (see **Table 1**). After confirming that the study subject met all inclusion and exclusion criteria, the sealed randomization envelope was opened and the subject was assigned to 1 of the 2 cohorts.

Because our center did not know which graft the subject would be randomized to before this, we were unable to preauthorize graft applications until after the randomization. Therefore, to neutralize any bias related to the lag phase of obtaining insurance authorization for graft placement, week 0 of the study was defined as the first week a biologic graft was placed on the study ulcer. On average, insurance

Table 1
Inclusion and exclusion criteria

Inclusion Criteria	Exclusion Criteria
• Able to give informed consent • Age 18 y or greater • Negative serum pregnancy test if subject of childbearing potential • VLU size >1 cm^2 and <40 cm^2 and <5 mm deep • VLU persisted >30 d despite medically supervised conventional wound care, including multilayer venous compression therapy • Ankle-brachial index >0.5 or biphasic or triphasic Doppler signals in the dorsalis pedis and posterior tibial arteries of the affected extremity	• Suspected gangrene or wound infection on any part of the affected limb • Hypersensitivity to bovine collagen or agarose (listed in Apligraf directions for use) • Hypersensitivity to any of the antibiotics or preservation agents (listed in the TheraSkin Instructions for use) • Subject previously treated in this clinical study • Subject has participated in another clinical trial involving a device or a systemically administered investigational study drug or treatment within 30 d of randomization visit • Subject is currently receiving (ie, within 30 d of randomization visit) or scheduled to receive a medication or treatment that, in the opinion of the investigator, known to interfere with or affect the rate of wound healing (eg, systemic steroids, immunosuppressive therapy, autoimmune disease therapy, cytostatic therapy within the 12 mo before randomization, dialysis, radiation therapy to the foot, vascular surgery, angioplasty or thrombolysis) • Subject has leg ulcers secondary to a disease other than venous ulcers (eg, vasculitis, neoplasm, or hematological disorders) • Subject has been treated with growth factors, engineered tissues, or skin substitutes within 30 d of randomization • Subject has a history of 1. Endstage renal disease 2. Immunosuppression 3. Severe malnutrition 4. Severe liver disease 5. Aplastic anemia 6. Scleroderma 7. Positive for AIDS or human immunodeficiency virus 8. Connective tissue disorder 9. Sickle cell anemia 10. Osteomyelitis 11. Bone cancer or metastatic disease of the affected limb 12. Irradiation of the affected extremity 13. Chemotherapy within the last 12 mo • Subject is employee or relative of any member of the investigational site or sponsor • Subject does not have health insurance

authorization took 1 to 2 weeks per subject. All subjects had to once again meet all the inclusion and exclusion criteria on the day the first graft was placed and throughout the 20 week study period. If a randomized subject was not qualified for insurance coverage, that subject would be discharged from the study but would continue to receive medical care as needed. In this case, the randomization envelope was also discarded and the next subject to be randomized was chosen by the next envelope in sequence.

Over the initial 12 weeks of the study, each subject received graft applications in accordance with manufacturer specifications. All wounds were evaluated at least weekly by the investigators, at which time they were measured, photographed, debrided, and grafted as needed. The subjects were followed until the study wound was completely healed (defined as 100% epithelialization without drainage) for up to 20 weeks.

All graft applications occurred during the first 12 weeks of the study only and were applied in accordance with manufacturer's recommendations. No grafts were used after week 12 in either cohort. Each subject was grafted weekly unless repeat grafts were contraindicated, based on clinical assessment (ie, infection) or if a graft was not available on the scheduled date of application. Grafting continued until wound healing occurred or until further grafts were not covered or authorized by the insurance carrier. After application, the grafts were covered with Mepilex transfer foam (Molnlycke Health Care, Norcross, GA, USA) or Adaptic (Systagenix, Quincy, MA, USA). Both cohorts received weekly dressing changes with a nonadherent contact layer of either Mepilex transfer foam or Adaptic and a multilayer compression dressing composed of either Kendall Kerlix (Medtronic, Minneapolis, MN, USA) and Coban (3M, St Paul, MN, USA), or Coban 2 Layer Compression system (3M, St Paul, MN, USA). Subjects who were highly exudative with strike-through were changed biweekly throughout the study. Standard multilayer compression dressings were used as adjunctive therapy over the primary dressing with all subjects throughout the study. Negative pressure wound therapy, lymphedema pump therapy, and local anesthetics for debridement were not used with any subject during the study.

Any wounds that failed to heal after the initial 12 weeks were treated for an additional 8 weeks with multilayer compression therapy alone and followed for delayed healing.

Demographics for each subject were recorded. These included age, gender, initial wound size, wound location, diabetes, body mass index (BMI), morbid obesity, peripheral vascular disease (PVD), malnutrition, daily smoking, daily alcohol use, lymphedema, and h/o neuropathy. PVD was assessed by examination, Doppler, ankle-brachial index, and noting any prior vascular disease history. Morbid obesity was defined as either subject weight greater than 100 lb greater than ideal body weight, BMI greater than or equal to 40, or BMI greater than or equal to 35 with obesity-related comorbidity. Malnutrition was defined as BMI less than or equal to 18.49.

Chi-squared analysis was performed to determine if there were any significant differences in the demographics of the 2 cohorts. Multivariate logistic regression analysis was used to evaluate individually recorded variables on the combined cohort data to determine what factors might impact wound closure. The Fisher exact test was used to compare healing rates between cohorts. The Welch 2-sample t-test was used to determine if there were significant differences in the number of grafts required to achieve closure. A power calculation was also performed to predict the risk of type 2 error. Critical endpoints were complete wound closure and time to wound closure.

All adverse events, treatment cessation, and study withdrawals were recorded. Serious adverse events were reported to the IRB.

RESULTS

There were 31 subjects enrolled and randomized into 1 of the 2 cohorts. There were 4 subjects who were randomized but then dropped out of the study. Of the subjects who did not complete the study, 3 subjects did not receive any grafts. Among the 3 subjects who did not receive any grafts, 1 was moved to a nursing home in another state within 2 weeks of randomization. The second subject failed to meet inclusion criteria during the period between insurance approval and scheduling of the first graft. The third subject was randomized but was found to no longer meet exclusion criteria before the first grafting was done. A fourth subject did receive the first Apligraf but was not compliant and was lost to follow-up immediately after graft placement. This left 27 subjects who completed the study, with 15 randomized to the TheraSkin cohort, and 12 randomized to the Apligraf cohort.

Table 2 describes the cohort demographics. The cohorts were equally matched with no significant differences in the demographics. Binary demographics are reported as a percentage and were evaluated with chi-squared statistical testing. Continuous variables were expressed as mean and standard deviation and evaluated with 2-sample t-testing. Normal probability plots on all continuous variables did not indicate any significant deviations from normality.

Multivariate logistic regression was conducted first individually on the recorded variables. For the combined cohort data, the baseline wound size was statistically significant with respect to the proportion of wounds healed ($P = .02815$).

The analysis of the study data focused on the percentage of wounds closed at 12 and 20 weeks, the number of grafts used, and the total cost of treatment in each cohort.

At 12 weeks, 93.3% (14/15) of the TheraSkin subjects experienced complete ulcer healing, whereas 75.0% (9/12) of the Apligraf subjects experienced complete healing. Although the healing rate at 12 weeks was higher in the TheraSkin cohort, there was no significant difference using the Fisher exact test (OR 0.227, $P = .294$).

At 20 weeks, 93.3% (14/15) of the TheraSkin subjects experienced complete ulcer healing, whereas 83.3% (10/12) of the Apligraf subjects experienced complete healing. Similarly, although the healing rate was higher at week 20 in the TheraSkin cohort, there was no significant difference using the Fisher exact test (OR 0.371, $P = .569$).

On average 2.27 grafts per subject (n 15) were used in the TheraSkin cohort, whereas 3.33 grafts per subject (n 12) were used in the Apligraf cohort. Although fewer grafts were needed to obtain complete epithelialization of the treated ulcers with the TheraSkin subjects than with the Apligraf subjects, no significant difference in the

Table 2
Cohort demographics

	Apligraf	TheraSkin	Chi-Squared Test	2-Sample t-Test
Age (y)	63.7 ± 13.4	66.3 ± 18.0	—	NSD $P = .672$
Gender	58.3% male	66.7% male	NSD $P = .655$	—
Initial wound size (cm^2)	6.37 ± 6.95	4.94 ± 4.43	—	NSD $P = .545$
Wound location	100% calf	100% calf	NSD $P = 1$	—
Diabetes	33.3%	46.7%	NSD $P = .696$	—
BMI	33.52 ± 9.91	36.63 ± 10.29	—	NSD $P = .4335$
Morbid obesity	50%	66.7%	NSD $P = .452$	—
PVD	8.3%	33.3%	NSD $P = .182$	—
Malnutrition (BMI ≤18.49)	0%	0%	NSD $P = 1$	—
Daily smoking	25%	6.7%	NSD $P = .294$	—
Daily alcohol	0%	0%	NSD $P = 1$	—
Lymphedema	8.3%	13.3%	NSD $P \sim 1$	—
Neuropathy	16.7%	13.3%	NSD $P \sim 1$	—

Abbreviation: NSD, no significant difference.

mean number of grafts needed between the 2 groups was found using the Welch 2-sample t-test ($P = .119$).

Using the Welsh 2-sample t-test, the average graft cost per subject in the TheraSkin cohort ($2495.33/subject) was significantly lower ($P = .0399$) than the average graft cost per subject in the Apligraf cohort ($4316.67/subject) (**Table 3**). The cost analysis was based solely on the cost of the biologic graft material because all other factors (eg, compression dressing, contact dressing, time required to apply) were the same between the 2 cohorts.

There were no adverse events related to the study. No subjects revoked their consent for the study after enrollment but 1 subject was lost to follow-up, as mentioned previously.

When the study ulcer was healed, no subjects returned to our wound healing center within 6 weeks of the study for any care related to the study ulcers.

A power calculation was performed with a 2-tail assessment and, assuming a standard deviation in healing rates of 30% in each group, with alpha equals 0.05, a power of only 35% was achieved. The data presented here would require at least 22 subjects in each cohort to achieve a power of 80%, assuming a standard deviation in healing rates of 30%.

DISCUSSION

With regard to design, this pilot study represents the first randomized prospective trial in which a head-to-head comparison between Apligraf and TheraSkin was used to examine outcomes for VLUs, in conjunction with compression therapy. As with all clinical studies, there are always shortcomings that may influence study outcome. The most significant factor is the power of the study. Because this is a pilot study, it was designed to give a general feel for the differences in performance of these 2 treatment options. Data from this study will likely be used to determine future study designs. Consequently, differences in closure rate were not statistically significant.

In this study, reapplication of grafts was scheduled to occur on a weekly basis; however, there were some inconsistencies because a graft could be skipped at the discretion of the investigators in some specific instances (ie, infection). Although the grafts were normally applied on a weekly basis, there were some occasions when they were applied less often.

VLU treatment includes compression as part of the standard of care. Although compression therapy was used here, it is typically very difficult to apply compression in exactly the same fashion from patient to patient and visit to visit. In some cases,

Table 3
Results

	Apligraf	TheraSkin	Statistical Test
VLU healing at 12 wk	75%	93.3%	Not significant Fisher exact test $P = .294$
VLU healing at 20 wk	83.3%	93.3%	Not significant Fisher exact test $P = .569$
Number of grafts per subject used	3.33	2.27	Not significant 2-sample t-test $P = .119$
Average cost per subject treated	$4316.67	$2495.33	Significant 2-sample t-test $P = .0399$

some patients received more than 1 compression dressing per week when the wound was particularly exudative. Additionally, some subjects had Mepilex, whereas others had Adaptic covering the graft, before application of the compression dressing. These inconsistencies may potentially represent an additional bias in the outcomes observed.

In this study, VLUs were treated with either TheraSkin or Apligraf in conjunction with compression therapy. Each graft was prepared and was applied in accordance with the respective manufacturers recommendations. Although wounds treated with TheraSkin closed at a slightly higher rate than wounds treated with Apligraf, this difference was not statistically significant. It is also noted that the slight difference in demographics of the subjects in each cohort was not statistically significant. The lack of statistical significance may be the result of the small sample size rather than a lack of a statistically significant difference in outcomes.

In both the TheraSkin and Apligraf cohorts, the closure rate was slightly better than in previous studies.[4,5] It is unclear why this difference exists but it may be attributable to the consistency of care provided, as well as that the average number of grafts applied was slightly more than the number reported in previous studies, in both groups. In addition, variations in wound sizes in each of these studies may also play a role in the closure rates.

Although there was no statistically significant difference in the rate of wound closure or the number of grafts applied to achieve closure, the average cost for treatment in each cohort was significantly different, which is attributed to the difference in actual costs of the 2 graft materials. Based on the limited data presented, the cost to treat with Apligraf was 42.2% greater than treatment with TheraSkin.

SUMMARY

In this study, the impact of 2 types of skin substitute grafts used for the treatment of VLUs was compared in a prospective, randomized fashion. The 2 cohorts were well-matched, both in size and demographics.

Although there were higher VLU healing rates with the TheraSkin cohort at both 12 weeks (93.3% vs 75.0%) and 20 weeks (93.3% vs 83.3%), these healing rate differences were not statistically significant. There was also no statistically significant difference in the number of grafts required to achieve closure owing to the small sample size presented.

There was a significant decrease in cost for the appropriate graft sizes needed to treat the study subjects in the TheraSkin cohort ($2495.33/subject) compared with the Apligraf cohort ($4316.67/subject), even though the initial wound sizes were not significantly different between groups.

Based on the data presented here, the use of either of these biologics in conjunction with compression therapy is a safe and effective way to treat VLUs. Although the cost of treatment associated with TheraSkin was lower, both products have demonstrated that they are more likely to help a patient achieve closure than just compression therapy alone.[4]

REFERENCES

1. Franks PJ, Barker J, Collier M, et al. Management of patients with venous leg ulcers: challenges and current best practice. J Wound Care 2016;25(Suppl 6):S1–67.
2. Hodde JP, Allam R. Small intestinal submucosa wound matrix for chronic wound healing. Wounds 2007;19(7):157–62.

3. Rice JB, Desai U, Cummings AK, et al. Burden of venous leg ulcers in the United States. J Med Econ 2014;17(5):347–56.
4. Falanga V, Margolis D, Alvarez O, et al. Rapid healing of venous ulcers and lack of clinical rejection with an allogeneic cultured human skin equivalent. Arch Dermatol 1998;134(3):293–300.
5. Landsman AS, Cook J, Cook E, et al. A retrospective clinical study of 188 consecutive patients to examine the effectiveness of a biologically active cryopreserved human skin allograft (TheraSkin®) on the treatment of diabetic foot ulcers and venous leg ulcers. Foot Ankle Spec 2011;4(1):29–41.
6. Kolluri R. Management of venous ulcers. Tech Vasc Interv Radiol 2014;17(2): 132–8.
7. Barber C, Watt A, Pham C, et al. Influence of bioengineered skin substitutes on diabetic foot ulcer and venous leg ulcer outcomes. J Wound Care 2008;17(12): 517–27.
8. Landsman A, Rosines E, Houck A, et al. Characterization of a cryopreserved split-thickness human skin allograft-TheraSkin. Adv Skin Wound Care 2016;29(9): 399–406.

Printed and bound by CPI Group (UK) Ltd, Croydon, CR0 4YY
07/10/2024
01040502-0012